Old Urologists Never Die…They Just Detumesce into Flaccidity

John McHugh

"Ye gods John! A urologist? Do you know what they do?"

Jennie Cooper Davis McHugh, single parent of five boys, upon hearing that her fourth son John, had chosen to go into urology.

Dedicated to:

Roy Witherington, MD
Arthur Smith, MD
Kenneth Lennox, MD

Medical College of Georgia

Urological Wit and Wisdom
John McHugh M.D.
Edited by David Rider
Special thanks to Travis Massey and Magic Craft Studio
Copyright © 2015 by Jennie Cooper Press
All rights reserved. No part of this book may be reproduced or transmitted in any form or by any means without written permission from the author.
ISBN-13: 978-0988661837
Cover picture by Jennie Cooper Davis McHugh (She obviously found humor in capturing my urgency incontinence and attempts at stemming it.)

Some of the anecdotal illustrations in this book are true to life and are included with the permission of the persons involved. All other illustrations are composites of real situations, and any resemblance to people living or dead is coincidental.

Unless otherwise referenced, all of the aphorisms, adages and sayings listed, I have heard, remembered or created over the years. It has been my experience that, because aphorisms express a general truth all of us have experienced, often times no definitive person can, for certain, be given the credit for its origin. This book concerns itself with illustrating aphorisms that have been meaningful to me throughout my career. Where there is a definitive author, I have so noted.

Prostate Cancer Blog-theprostatedecision.wordpress.com
Twitter-www.twitter.com/prostatediaries
LinkedIn-Linkedin.com/e/fpf/78723873
Email-info@ngurology.com
Available on Amazon.com, Createspace.com and Barnesandnoble.com
Are you an aphorist or know an aphorism you would like to share? Email it to me for Volume II.

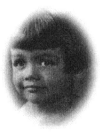

Jennie Cooper Press

"Calm as a Hurricane"

Urological Wit and Wisdom

101 Aphorisms, Adages and Illustrations for the Resident and Nascent Physician

John C. McHugh M.D.

I will not cut for stone even for patients in whom the disease is manifest; I will leave this operation to be performed by practitioners, specialists in this art.

The Hippocratic Oath

Table of Contents

"A Little More Than You Paid For"

Foreword

My mother loved to use old adages as aids to imparting advice as life's learning experiences arose. Although "the pot calling the kettle black," "it's going to be too wet to plough," and "you can lead a horse to water but you can't make him drink," were commonly called upon, I believe "a little knowledge is a dangerous thing" was her favorite. She reminded me of the saying so many times that as I got older, she only needed to say, "a little knowledge John" with a sarcastic upward inflection in her voice, and I knew what she meant.
From *The Decision*

There is a very fine line between the nuances of an aphorism, an adage, a truism, a maxim, an axiom, or a saying. It is the aphorism, however, which has been most associated with the medical profession. William Osler used concise sentences that embodied the essence of a particular facet of the art of Medicine. Over time his aphorisms, as well as those of others, have been passed down in medical schools, residency programs, and in private practice.

My first exposure to aphorisms, although at the time I did not know that they were called that, was during my residency. Just as I loved my mother's sayings, so too, I particularly enjoyed the use of them in my urological residency by the various attendings. My favorite one of all was, "Don't buy shoes in the morning and don't pull tubes at night." It is perfect; it's terse, to the point, it speaks volumes to the management of tubes, drains, and catheters and expresses a general urological truth that one can easily identify.

As you read what follows, you'll note that you have heard most of the aphorisms, and you'll also remember an occasion where it applied. You'll probably smile and acknowledge at some point in your career, or even on a reoccurring basis, these sayings have applied to situations familiar to you.

Now about giving credit where credit is due. I distinctly remember Dr. Witherington telling me about "Every physician should have a top hat and a case of hemorrhoids; the first for an air of distinction and the second for that look of concern" and I have since seen that saying attributed to others. It is my feeling that the vast majority of these aphorisms, except those specifically attributed to someone like Osler, has been handed down through time and have been altered. I have, however, listed several books that I perused, but all of the aphorisms, adages, and illustrations, unless otherwise noted, are from my memory and personal experiences. By listing them I am in no way taking credit for them. Also, although some have a urological slant, all of these sayings and illustrations can easily apply across the various specialties of medicine.

My wife had recommended to me to do a hundred and one, but as I got going the sayings, phrases, aphorisms, truisms, and experiences just ballooned ad infinitum. Over several months I kept a running list of aphorisms on a sheet of paper I taped to a door way in our clinic. Seeing patients throughout the course of each day made me recall these sayings in a steady stream. The well never went dry. I am stopping at one hundred and twenty five, but I am continuing the list for the next volume. I have had way too much fun with this project.

I hope you enjoy this collection and that maybe there will be one or two of these you have not heard and will use yourself. For the patient or student, an aphorism helps explain a disease. For the colleague, an aphorism is similar to a secret handshake: it's a concept that all medical personnel can easily identify because of a common experience that embodies it.

This book is dedicated to my attendings in urology while I was at the Medical College of Georgia. Most of the aphorisms listed I probably heard first from one of them. No attempt has been made to attach every aphorism to a person. In addition to the wonderful training I received as the result of these men, the greatest gifts they gave me were the aphorisms.

Dr. "W," it's been almost thirty years, and, like a prostate, I too have just about vine ripened.

John McHugh

"The examining physician often hesitates to make the necessary examination because it involves soiling the finger."

William Mayo

1

Don't Buy Shoes in the Morning, and Don't Pull Tubes at Night

Putting aside the givens and prerequisites of a good physician– empathy, integrity, skill, and intelligence – there is also a lot of strategy involved. We all know the caring physician who spends time with his patients, however full his waiting room is of patients who have been waiting for hours. We know the surgeon who is well liked and does a decent enough job, but is slow as molasses doing procedures that others do much quicker. So what is it? Is it time management? Is it prioritizing? Is it knowing when to "fish or cut bait?" Is it knowing the mind of your patient? Or is it knowing your strengths and weaknesses, learning from experience, and listening to the advice of those who have come before you? Is it intuitive or could it be strategy? Good doctors minimize the "noise."

In many ways, *The Art of War* by Sun Tzu applies to the physician's management of the cards he is dealt throughout his day. Think of yourself as preparing for battle with your enemies, that being the patient, the disease, time, or even your colleagues. Keep in mind some of the tenants outlined by Tzu:

"If you know neither the enemy nor yourself, you will succumb in every battle."

"Strategy without tactics is the slowest route to victory. Tactics without strategy is the noise before defeat."

"The supreme art of war is to subdue the enemy without fighting."

Rule: You can control your practice of medicine, or you can let it control you. Your decisions should be made in such a way that in the event of an adverse consequence, it favors you and at a time of your choosing. Repeat after me: "Don't pull tubes at night."

"In all arts and sciences both the end the means should be equally in our control."-Aristotle

2

Primum non Nocoere: First, Do No Harm

When I was a urological resident at the Medical College of Georgia, I had an interaction with one of the attendings during a stint at the VA hospital. I was a chief resident and, as all budding surgeons do, I was looking for cases to hone my surgical skills. As a urological resident the good cases were usually something rare like a pediatric hypospadias repair, a radical prostatectomy or cystectomy (a cystectomy being the crème de la crème of the urologist's playbook).

On one occasion, I had a patient whose prostate biopsy came back positive and, having been given the options, wanted to have the prostate removed. The patient was overweight with the predominance of his weight around were the prostatectomy incision would be made. With the patient lying on the exam table, I step out to get the attending, make my case for a prostatectomy, and then bring him back to meet the patient. After giving the details of the biopsy the attending says, "Well John, let's meet this gentleman."

We go to the exam room door, and as I open the door no more than six inches, the attending catches a glimpse of my patient's protuberant silhouette and profile on the table. He places his hand on mine, stops the motion of the door, and closes the door.

He then looks at me very seriously and says, "No way in hell, John!" It was exactly the right thing to say and a teachable moment.

Rule: You are supposed to make people better not worse. Think about it ahead of time. Fat is the mud of surgery.

"No operation should be carried out unless absolutely necessary ... nor should a surgeon operate unless he would undergo the same operation himself in similar circumstances." -John Hunter

"Whenever a doctor cannot do good, he must be kept from doing harm." -Hippocrates

3
God Must Have Been a Urologist

There was an attending at the Medical College who had cholangitis and almost died. Directly over his head and behind his desk was a framed saying regarding God being a urologist. I think urology must piss off other surgical subspecialties for this very reason. After all, it isn't fair.

Why are there two kidneys and only one gallbladder? And why are there two testicles and only one pancreas? Why does a hot appendix need to be operated on at once and ureteral stones can wait until the morning if there is no fever and the pain is controlled? Most stones, bladder tumors, and symptoms of prostate enlargement can be managed endoscopically without an incision. Prostate cancer and kidney cancer are well suited to robotic removal. Vasectomies take less than fifteen minutes and can be done on an exam table with oral sedation. With the advent of Doppler ultrasound, torsion of the testicle, which used to be the "appendix of the urologist," now is easily detectable.

So what is it? Why doesn't everyone choose to be a urologist? Few emergencies, increasing patient population and innovative, minimally-invasive modalities all would be evidence for choosing this surgical subspecialty. Urology is gentleman's surgery. And of course there is the two kidneys thing.

Well, it's the penis. Urology takes a special person. The penis intimidates. A urologist has to be earthy and must have thick rugae, well, skin. Even our signature diagnostic maneuver, the rectal, is an exam the patient doesn't want and one most physicians can easily be persuaded not to do.

When I told my mother that I had decided to be a urologist she said, "Ye Gods John! Do you know what they do?"

"Why couldn't you be a surgeon?" she said.

Rule: You probably have to comfortable saying the word "penis" in mixed company if you want to be a urologist.

"The chief function of a consultant is to make a rectal examination that you have omitted."- Osler

4
I Love Breasts, John

My wife and I were at a party for an end of the year tennis celebration. I was standing in a circle of women and the subject of plastic surgery came up. As I often do, I related a story regarding a good friend of mine who is a plastic surgeon. This friend had initially planned to be a neurosurgeon and changed to general surgery. After that he decided to be a plastic surgeon which required another two years of fellowship training. We were talking one day, and I asked him how he had settled on plastic surgery.

"Well John," he said, "I love breasts."

I love telling that story and it always gets a good laugh. After this telling with this particular group, however, there was a comment from one of the women in the circle which was not only clever but also hits at the subliminal thought process of how people view urologists.

"So, tell us John. Why then, did you choose urology?"

Rule: It is easier to say you are a plastic surgeon than a urologist; and, you get to work on better anatomy.

Will Mayo, one of the founders of the Mayo Clinic, visited Johns Hopkins and observed Dr. Halsted perform a radical mastectomy. It is said that Will stepped out of the operating room shaking his head after 2 hours and said: "My God, this is the first time I have seen the wound healing at the upper end while it is still being operated upon at the lower end."-Peter D. Olch

I had not had a rectal exam since medical school. (It had been performed on me by a fellow female medical student twenty years previously as part of an introductory class on physical exams. I distinctly remember not having had the opportunity of returning the favor of performing a breast exam on her.) From The Decision.

"She got her good looks from her father - he`s a plastic surgeon."-Groucho Marx

5
The Money Spends Well

I t goes without fail that during performing a vasectomy the young male, in an awkward attempt to make conversation, invariably asks the question: "So, doc, what made you want to go into this profession?"

Of course this question is posed while I am in the process of manipulating the scrotum to identify the vas deferens. As tempted as I am to say something inappropriate, I will usually relate that I have never liked call, and that the urologic residency program in Augusta did not require a hospital call as the other surgical residencies did. I remember learning this fact from a friend who had elected to pursue urology and at that moment I decided to be a urologist.

Well, as much grief as I have received about being a urologist, it did not dawn on me that my wife, too, might be subject to this type of questioning. Sure enough I witnessed it at a gathering, and I must say my wife handled it quite well.

"Karen, what's it like being married to a urologist?"

"The money spends well," she responded.

"John, how much do you urologists charge to just hold down that ESWL button?" A petty and jealous colleague asks.
"First of all, I don't hold down the button. Second of all, in answer to your sarcastic question, a lot," I tell him.

Rule: Don't defend a position. Embrace it and give it right back to 'em.

Years ago I was in the doctor's lounge and a radiation therapist came in to get a cup of coffee. An internal medicine doctor accosted him shortly after he entered and asked sarcastically, "How much do you charge for hospital paid technicians to use machines to treat your patients?"

Without a pause the reply came, probably hearing this type of drivel before, "Tell me about your lab over there at your clinic; what do you charge? We all have our gimmicks."

6
No Good Deed Goes Unpunished

Years ago I was treating a prominent public figure in our community for kidney stones. The offending stone was in the renal pelvis, and its characteristics were best suited for a percutaneous nephrostolithotomy. His schedule was such that he asked that the procedure be done on a Saturday.

"I'll be forever grateful," he said.

I was not on call that weekend, however, I arranged for the surgical team to be there to include the interventional radiologist. The case in radiology to place the nephrostomy began at 7:30. At around 10:30, and after all of the surgical team had waited three hours for what should have taken thirty minutes, we receive word that he was unable to place a nephrostomy. This in turn meant that the case could not be done, making the whole morning a waste for everyone.

I am left with the task of informing the patient about the difficulties of nephrostomy placement, that this type of thing occurs commonly, and that we might attempt another day and maybe with a different radiologist.

The patient was disappointed, but I felt at the time that he was appropriate and understanding. Although we arranged a follow-up visit, he did not keep his appointment. I did not see him again until years later; I believe it was in a restaurant. I noticed him and asked about whatever came of the stone he had.

"Oh, I went to Atlanta and had it done by people who knew what they were doing."

Rule: Don't stray far from the usual routine. It rarely pays off. Treat your family and friends as you would your regular patients. As Dr. Dick Treat used to say, "We do it the same way every time."

"Do not judge confreres by the reports of patients, well meaning, perhaps, but often strangely and sadly misrepresenting."-Osler

7
People Talk

I had just become the Chief Resident in Urology and we were making evening rounds with a new batch of interns and residents. As it turned out, one of the new interns was in our urology program. He had to do the prerequisite two years of general surgery before moving into urology and happened to be rotating through the urology service. He was a Citadel graduate, which piqued my interest, as I was in the cadet ROTC program at North Georgia College in Dahlonega. The very first patient we come to during rounds was scheduled for a TURP the next morning. During rounds, I tell the urology intern to be sure the chart was up to date and to have a permit signed for the procedure.

"You do it. You're doing the procedure," he said.

I must say he looked good saying that. He must have thought he had made advancements for national intern rights.

"May I speak to you out here for a minute?" I asked, leaving the others in the patient's room.

"Your next rotation I believe is on vascular surgery, and after that ENT, and then orthopedics. I am friends with all the chief residents on those and all of the other services which you will be on over the next two years."

After a pause, I added, "People talk. Has what I have said to you made sense?"

"Yes, it does," he said. "I'll get the chart in order."

Rule: What goes around comes around. To get along you have to get along.

"Look wise, say nothing, and grunt. Speech was given to conceal thought."-Osler

8

The Well Wear a Crown Only the Sick Can See

I was asked to see a quadriplegic patient in anticipation of placing a suprapubic tube. The patient was a nice enough fellow. He had a lot of questions, and, at times, I felt he was suspicious of my intentions. I picked up on his demeanor, and, as it was late in the day, I was a bit annoyed by him and really didn't like his attitude. I mean, I was there to help. When it came to dealing with doctors this was not his first rodeo.

I ask if I can examine the lower abdomen area, and he consents. I pull his blanket down to his upper thighs. A catheter is indwelling. The penis has the usual bullous edema, and there is the smell of urine. His legs are atrophic, and his arms are motionless by his side.

After examining the suprapubic area, I pull the blanket and sheets back up and tell him that he appears to be a good candidate for the procedure. I explained what I'd be doing and answered all of his questions. I turn to leave and am at the doorway when the patient calls to me.

"Can you fix my blanket better under my chin?"

"Sure," I say.

I had replaced the blanket back to where I thought I'd found it. It had been under his shoulders on each side and then up underneath the chin to a particular place. With some effort and adjustment we were get it back exactly like it was and how he wanted it. I remember thinking at the time, "He sure is being picky."

After leaving, my mind went back to when I was an orderly in college. I worked at the West Georgia Medical Center in my hometown of LaGrange, Georgia. I was on a rotational schedule, which meant that each morning I would go to the head nurse's office and get my assignment. More often than not, I was sent to the paraplegic/stroke wing in the older portion of the hospital. My job would be to give baths all day. I also would shave patients if they desired. For some reason, that area of Georgia had a large number of men that had suffered spinal injuries from pulp wood work. In the course of the baths, I learned a lot about these patients, their previous life and how they happened to be where they were. Many knew my grandfather, Robert Cooper Davis, a pharmacist.

Every so often, I'd be bathing a patient and they would not cooperate with me. It would be little things, but it made my job much harder. They might prevent me from moving their head from left to right thereby preventing me from shaving them completely. I remember getting mad at them and forcing the head to the necessary position. I would talk to them in threatening tones.

"I am going to shave you whether you like it or not, so you might as well not fight me on this."

To them it was almost like a game. Maybe they were exerting some semblance of control, something they did not otherwise have in their particular predicament.

These memories of the past and what had just happened with the suprapubic patient then hit me as being very similar occurrences. Can you imagine what these patients have been through? What these conditions and injuries had done to their self-esteem? I am sorry, but these patients get a pass.

Rule: If a quadriplegic wants a blanket a certain way, and it will probably be that way for hours because he has no control to change it, then make it that way.

"Let me be sick myself if sometimes the malady of my patient be not a disease to me."-Sir Thomas Browne

"To you the silent workers of the ranks, in villages and country districts, in the slums of our large cities, in the mining camps and factory towns, in the homes of the rich, and in the hovels of the poor, to you is given the harder task of illustrating with your lives the Hippocratic standards of Learning, of Sagacity, of Humanity, and of Probity."-Osler

"Wherever the art of medicine is loved, there is also the love of humanity." -Hippocrates

9
If It Ain't Broke, Don't Fix It

So you are seeing one of the most difficult clinical problems in urology today, that being the little old lady who has total incontinence.

"If I feel the urge, I better get there quickly."

"Do you leak with coughing or sneezing?"

"I don't sneeze. I do leak with coughing and getting out of the car."

"How about just walking around? Does urine just come down without warning?"

"Yes, and I wear five pads a day."

"Did the medicine I gave you help at all?"

"Yes. I am not cured, but I have improved enough that I can live with my current level of leaking."

Okay. This is where the finesse comes in. Sure, you could talk to this patient about adding another medicine, say Tofranil to complement the Vesicare to improve the urgency component. Sure, you could mention a bulking agent or a sling for the ISD, but the patient has told you, "I can live with my current level of leaking."

Leave it at that until the patient asks for something else to be done. More medicines or more procedures in a patient who states she is content will only complicate matters and worse yet, make things worse.

Rule: Let the patient be the judge of what they are content with, and leave them alone. The enemy of good is better. About the picture below...well maybe that does need "fixin."

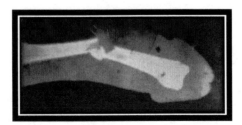

10
The Power of "I don't know."

Patients ask a lot of questions. Not all do, and some ask more than others. Some ask a different question while you are answering the question that was just asked. Some ask questions based on something that happened to a friend or what another doctor told them. Some ask good questions that help the situation at hand and some ask questions just to get their money's worth.

I have a neurologist friend who, as the patient begins to fire up the questions, cuts them off and says, "Sir. I have five questions for you. If you answer my five questions it will allow me to help you."

How my friend conducts his office visit may sound rude to you. However, if I see a thousand kidney stones a year, I know what is important in the history that will determine the treatment options. Doesn't it make sense for me to conduct the interview in a succinct manner directed toward the disease process? Do we need to know what the patient was doing when the pain hit or what a friend did when he had a stone? What if you can't break the question cycle, and you have already used the telling your nurse to knock on the door in five minutes trick?

At the appropriate time you simply answer the question with, "I don't know." This is so simplistic it is brilliant. It will stun the patient and break the question cycle, as every question with an answer begets fodder for another question. It has to end somewhere. You will be viewed as thoughtful, and their problem will seem unique and difficult. This all works in your favor.

At this point you quickly ask your questions, state your treatment plan, and stand up. These actions send the message that the visit is approaching its conclusion.

Rule: You are the expert. You know the answers you need to treat the problem, the patient doesn't. Direct, teach, and treat them with empathy. Osler said it was okay to say, "Perhaps."

Sydenham was called "a man of many doubts," and therein lay the secret of his great strength.-Osler

11

When You Hear Hoof Beats Think Horses, Not Zebras

M en commonly complain of the lack of energy, decreased libido and deterioration of their erections. Certainly the cause of this triad is often multifactorial; often times these symptoms prompt the urologist to obtain a serum testosterone. There might even be an inquiry as to recent changes in medications, relationships, or at work. Other medical conditions, such as vascular disease or diabetes, come quickly to mind. All of these possibilities are reasonable hypotheses' for any urologist. But what if the doctor ordered a brain CT to rule out a prolactin producing pituitary tumor? Considering that the average, practicing urologist might see this condition only five times in a career, this diagnostic study and the inconvenience and expense it entails, can be saved for a later time after the other more common, and much more likely, concerns play out.

The term "Zebra" was coined in the 1940's by Dr. Theodore Woodward of the Maryland School of Medicine and means an unusual or rare diagnosis. These should be considered and pursued only after the more common etiologies have been evaluated. Common sense, huh?

Rule: Urethritis is more likely to be related to taking baths with a new bubble bath then Reiter's Syndrome. Changing bathing habits is a much more cost effective diagnostic maneuver than a multispecialty workup.

"Queer cases" are usually abnormal types of common conditions.

12
Common Things Occur Commonly

My kidneys hurt right here," the patient says as he is rubbing the palm of his hand horizontally across the lower back from one side all the way to the other. The grimaced facial expression complements the hand movement, and, in unison, it is a picture of distress.

"My doctor saw blood in my urine and sent me here for a kidney stone," the patient says.

"Does it hurt if you bend or stoop?"

"Yes."

"Does it hurt worse when you get up in the morning and somewhat improves as you move around?"

"Yes."

"The pain you have is real. Our job is to see if it is urological or not. You may not have a stone."

"If it is not a stone then where is the pain coming from?"

"It may be the muscles of your back."

"Where is the blood coming from then?"

"It may be coming from the prostate and unrelated to your pain which, as I said, is real, but may not be from a stone. We will order a CT scan and this study will confirm the diagnosis. In the meantime it is reasonable to give you something for pain."

Rule: Musculoskeletal back pain is more common than having kidney stone, and you can't reproduce stone pain with motion. In golf a slice will listen to you, but a hook won't hear a damn thing you say. Ureteral colic is a hook.

"Think of common diseases first."

13
All Bleeding Stops Eventually

For years, some friends and I went out west to fly fish and hike. The usual routine was a bush plane would drop us off at a dirt landing strip near a river, and then a week later pick us up some fifty miles or so up or down the river. This particular trip was in the Bob Marshall Wilderness in Montana on the Flathead River.

One day, a friend and I had hiked about two miles from the camp and then dropped down off the trail to a pretty run of the river. The plan was to fish the river back up to an area near the campsite and then return by the trail. In the process of fishing my friend cut his calf on an exposed and sharp branch from a fallen tree. There was immediate and profuse bleeding that was very concerning to my friend and somewhat to me. It was clear that it was superficial and that there was no arterial component to the injury. He took off his shorts, tore his boxers into a tourniquet and then asked me what I thought.

"It looks ok to me. Your boxers seem to have done the trick," I say.

He puts his pants back on sans boxers and we begin to fish again in the river. After about thirty minutes the underwear tourniquet is soaked in blood. Briefly peeking under the tourniquet, it still did not seem to me that it was a major injury. You know the old urology adage: "A teaspoon of blood in a gallon of water looks a lot more than it is."

"John, this looks pretty soaked to me. Is it going to be ok? I mean is this thing going to stop bleeding?"

"All bleeding stops... eventually," I respond.

"Thanks John. That is reassuring."

Rule: We made it back to camp and my friend, a lawyer, made it back alive to civilization as well unfortunately. The difference between a dead lawyer and raccoon on the highway: the raccoon has skid marks in front of it.

"The only weapon with which the unconscious patient can immediately retaliate upon the incompetent surgeon is hemorrhage."- William Stewart Halsted

14
Do You Have a Ruler?

One of my all-time favorite musicians is James Taylor. I discovered him in the early seventies and have seen him live on many occasions. Did you know he was originally signed by Apple Records? "Mudslide Slim and the Blue Horizon" is the first album I had by him, and it is absolutely a classic. All of the songs are iconic. The beginning of one of the songs goes, "I know this isn't a time for levity, but have you heard the story about Machine Gun Kelly?"

Being a urologist often lends itself to levity. Let me give you an example. There was a junior resident of mine, with whom I was close, who was called to the heart room to place a catheter. By the way, this is the perfect situation for urologic levity. You can imagine the scene; all the thoracic surgeons are there, along with the operating room staff. The paraphernalia of the cardiac pump team all brought to a standstill because they can't insert a catheter; the absolutely perfect set up to the comedic urologist to work his craft for the captive crowd assembled.

Well, they pull back the drape and there it is, in all its splendor, an appendage as the resident later described, "as long as from my forefinger to my elbow and the girth of my wrist." As the area was prepped for the procedure, the operating room scrub nurse asked what he will need to place the catheter.

"Do you need the filiforms, the Van Burens, a coude catheter, or cystoscope? What size catheter do you want?" she asked, having some urologic expertise.

"I want a ruler," he said. "I want to measure this thing!"

Rule: Sometimes a scientist must have facts to give credibility to the story. Men historically oversize things.

"Don't trust your memory. Make notes. Write down your observations."-Osler

15
Tomorrow Has Its Own Problems

There are many elements to being successful in medicine. Certainly, you must be ethical, work hard, and do good work. A quality that may well be overlooked by most practicing physicians is time management. But first, you guessed it, a story.

I was a junior resident, and on this particular night the attending on call was a private urologist at University Hospital in Augusta. I was seeing a patient in the emergency room that had been involved in a car accident and had an expanding renal hematoma. There were no other significant injuries. I don't remember the details of what happened precisely, but that is not important to the story. I spoke to the chief resident and then to the private on-call attending. When it was determined that the conservative measures were not the order of the day and after several phone conversations, it was decided to transfer the patient from Talmadge to University Hospital for surgery that night. As I recall, this was an unusual scenario, but deemed necessary considering the factors at play.

As if it were yesterday, I remember what the private urologist said to me that night when the decision was made to transfer and operate on the patient.

"Dr. McHugh, tomorrow has its own problems."

How true it is. He knew that he had two surgeries of his own the next morning and another 10 patients to see in the office. Temporizing with blood transfusions and putting off the inevitable would have only disrupted the entire next day. And there is no way of knowing what new stuff comes in from the emergency room or from add-ons from the office. You'd rather not operate at night, but when taking the long view, decisions are made with the above considerations in mind.

Rule: Why put off until tomorrow that which can be done today?

"Now the way of life that I preach is a habit to be acquired gradually by long and steady repetition. It is the practice of living for the day only, and for the day's work."
-Osler

16
The Tincture of Time

You, of course, have heard the saying that "wisdom comes with age." And, might I add that age and experience gives perspective. One who has practiced the art of urology for many years, and for that matter any specialty, begins to cultivate the skill of clairvoyance. Not only is it a skill but, better yet, a sense of how things will play out; something that only experience can give. I mention this to the young physician to admonish them to listen to their older colleagues. If an older physician advises you about a condition or type of patient, it would be my advice to consider that heavily in your treatment plan.

So this is where "tincture of time" comes in. Your older partner, or even you with time and experience, can see the whole process of a disease play out in your mind's eye from the get go. Think about a prostate biopsy pathology report showing elements of Gleason's 9. We know how that is going to end. As a young physician or surgeon, and family members of the patient, the first reaction to certain problem one might encounter is to take action; to do something. Order a test, get a consult, operate, give additional meds, etc. etc. etc.

What if, and I mean just *what if*, you have seen this scenario before and you have a feel that doing nothing and letting the "tincture of time" work its magic is the solution. Wouldn't that be better? Trust me, it is.

"A prudent physician will recommend the bark of the Quinquina when the patient would be obliged to eat the whole tree."

Rule: If doing nothing will work, then isn't that better than attempting to do something that might make matters worse?

"The young physician starts life with twenty drugs for each disease, and the old physician ends life with one drug for twenty diseases."-Osler

"To do nothing is also a good remedy."-Hippocrates

17

Once You Operate You Own Them

Y ou know the difference don't you? I mean, having a patient on your service that someone else operated on and handling *their* complication vs. someone on your service *you* operated on and handling your own complications. There is a big difference, my friend. Put simply, the former person is the good guy. Don't be the bad guy.

I learned this as a first-year urology resident. Of course, the mindset then was to jump at any opportunity to do surgery you had not done yet. I remember a patient that had a suprapubic prostatectomy at an outlying hospital and was sent to us because he would not stop bleeding. He had a suprapubic tube in place, a foley, and a midline, lower-abdominal incision. On arrival, the man was bleeding at each of these places. The solution is something surgical, right? Maybe take a look cystoscopically to fulgurate a bleeding point, or open the incision to find something to tie it off, right? The attending suggested doing more of the same– irrigation through the SP tube and out the foley, blood transfusions, and observation. We had started a drug, Amicar, which had a mile-long list of complications. Then we had the pharmacy mix up a solution of Alum and irrigated that into the suprapubic tube. This helped the bleeding, but was associated with intractable bladder spasms. B and O suppositories were added to the regimen.

After about a week, someone suggested we put the foley on tension, as well as on suction. Serial hemoglobins and the evaluation of the clotting factors were done. Each day on rounds, we recounted what we had done and then what other tricks we could do short of surgery. And then something unusual happened; the patient stopped bleeding. All the tubes were removed, and he went home.

Rule: Experience allows a surgeon, at reasonable odds, to know when it is better not to intervene surgically. Five year surgical program: The first year learning to operate and the last four learning when not to. "*When the primary indication for an operation is pain, that's what you'll get.*"-Mark M. Ravitch

18
If a Female Points "Right Here"

Back in the day, urologists did a whole lot of urethral dilations. They did them on children at the drop of a hat and for any urinary symptom from enuresis to dysuria. In fact, when I first started practice in 1986, the only referrals I got from pediatricians were to dilate a young male's urethra for a variety of voiding symptoms. As this required anesthesia, it wasn't long before, even though the patient was sent for me to do this specific procedure, I stopped agreeing with it and performing it. They soon stopped sending me those patients. It was then that I came to grips with the notion that, "I'm the urologist" send me a problem and I'll decide what is best from a urological perspective, not you."

As it pertains to women, I have had hundreds share horror stories of having been dilated in the office by an insensitive urologist. Based on my population of patients, it seems to me that urologists of old did urethral dilation on patients with difficult problems to discourage the patient from complaining any more. Much like one of the older urology attending's recommending SQ injection of 10% alcohol for the child with enuresis. I have seen urologists, because of their frustration in treating unrelenting and intractable bladder symptoms, prescribe three months of antibiotics to the female with IC, just so they wouldn't come back.

We still do urethral dilations of women for a myriad of issues, and it is beneficial for some. The ones that it helps swear by it.

How do you tell if they will be the person who will benefit? What I have found is that in the description of the symptom the patient will take a finger and point, sometimes touch, the urethra.

"It hurts right here."

Rule: If a female points to, or better yet touch, the urethra, they will benefit from urethral dilation.

19
The Doting Wife

The patient and wife are in the exam room holding hands when I enter. The complaint is erectile dysfunction unresponsive to medicines or injections. They had already been around the block and knew they wanted a penile prosthesis. After a discussion of the downside of the procedure the surgery is scheduled.

In the hospital the wife did not leave the patient's side, or, for that matter, the room. It seemed to me at the time that their relationship was either true love or bordering on being hokey; it was a bit too syrupy for me.

The patient did well with the surgery and I made an appointment for two weeks later to check on the incision. I told him he would be able to use the prosthesis in a month, and that at follow up I'd show him the inflation process.

In the office at the follow up visit, uncharacteristically, the patient is alone, and relates that he has done well. The incision is clean and healing appropriately.

"So, things look good. In two weeks you can come in and I'll show you how to cycle the prosthesis up and down and you can start using it."

"Oh doc, I've already used it several times. It works great, just don't tell my wife!"

Rule: Relationships can be tricky. Basically, you do what works. Who are we to judge? Prosthesis warranty: Five years or 50,000 strokes.

"Idleness is the mother of lechery; and a young man will find that absorption in any pursuit will do much to cool passions which, though natural and proper, cannot in the exigencies of our civilization always obtain natural and proper gratification." "Carnal concupiscence may be cooled and quelled-hard work of body and hard work of mind."-Osler

"One should always be in love. That is the reason one should never marry."
-Oscar Wilde

20
When It Comes To Edema the Scrotum Is the First to Know

I dare say that one of the most common consults a urologist will get throughout a career is the swollen testicles issue. Usually, it is an older male with multiple medical problems who is on the medical, farthest away from where the urology floor is.

When appraising the patient's room, everything on the surface appears, for the most part, normal. You see a foley emanating out from the patient and down to the collection device.

It is not until one pulls back the sheets do you see the problem: the swollen scrotum. Although the consult is for swollen testicles, it is clear to the trained eye that this issue is that old trusted friend of the urologist: the scrotum.

On further inspection, the urologist will see pedal edema that extends up into the thigh area, and yes, it is pitting indeed. Whether the patient is circumcised or not, but it is more prominent if he is not, the edema has engulfed the penis, and now the head is not recognizable. It is clear that whoever put in the foley had some degree of luck finding the meatus and the urologist is glad he was not called for the catheter insertion.

On palpation the edema is bullous in nature and despite vigorous manipulation of the testicles, which cannot be palpated for any anatomic purpose but only for tenderness; there is no reaction by the patient of pain. A scrotal ultrasound will confirm the benign nature of this condition, but is not necessary. Elevation of the scrotum on a rolled sheet is the treatment, but you order a scrotal ultrasound anyway for show.

Rule: The scrotum is a harbinger of fluid status, an innocent bystander in a bigger problem and correction of the edema elsewhere will resolve the scrotal issue. The scrotum is only trying to help the medical doctor.

Bullous edema of the scrotum: There will be no pain with vigorous manipulation of the testes.

21
Concatenation of Shadows

I was looking at an X-ray with a radiologist one time and noted an odd configuration that did not resemble a stone or bowel gas, but it was definitely something.

"What is this?" I ask.

"That, John, is a concatenation of shadows," he says.

In other words, he did not know what in the hell it was. He knew it was not bad. He knew what the bad things looked like and that wasn't one of them.

When I think of what that radiologist said, I think about difficult patients. I think about being a so called specialist. The difficult patient with the myriad of symptoms that contradict and point nowhere is very much like an X-ray with a concatenation of shadows.

As a specialist, you don't necessarily need to know what it is, but rather, what it is not. Knowing what it is not then begins the most difficult and arduous task of pursuing a diagnosis of exclusion. This is frustrating to the patient and physician alike, but does move the process forward.

Recently, I saw an older patient who was status post external beam radiation for prostate cancer. He was seen because said he felt his prostate had grown to the point of "closing off my bowels." I have never seen that in my entire career. Maybe once, in a very locally advanced prostate cancer case with concentric involvement of the rectum, the patient may have had some resultant bowel symptoms. This patient's gland and rectal area on exam, however, was essentially normal and he was referred back to the general physician to explore gastrointestinal etiologies for his symptoms.

Rule: You may not know what the diagnosis is, but experience helps you know what it is not and in turn takes a shade or two of gray off the concatenation of shadows that is your patient's diagnosis.

"Wisdom is the daughter of experience."-Leonardo da Vinci

22
Pain at the Tip of the Penis Think Prostate or Distal Stone

The penis in and of itself rarely hurts. Usually, if a patient tells you his penis hurts at rest, then it is probably a manifestation of an issue elsewhere.

Of course, when the patient complains about pain at the tip of the penis, an exam should ensue. Meatits, or some other irritation of penis, could be present. But the chief complaint is typically dysuria rather than pain with meatits.

A distal stone or prostatitis is most commonly the etiology, but convincing the patient of this is sometimes difficult. The concept of referred pain is not easily understood, and this is complicated by the lay person worrying that penile symptoms of any etiology are venereal related. A rash on the arm is eczema but if the same rash is on the penis it is something he caught. In the case of prostatitis, the prostate is tender on exam. If the patient adds that there is painful ejaculation, then the diagnosis is secure.

A distal stone in the area of the UVJ will cause dysuria, hematuria, and bladder symptoms most commonly, but also can manifest as discomfort at the tip of the penis. Women with distal stones are sometimes treated for weeks by the gynecologist for a refractory UTI before a CT confirms the diagnosis.

Rule: If the complaint is penile pain, then something's up. And it is not the penis, *per se.*

*"My penis hurts" "You have a ureteral stone." "Why does my penis hurt; shouldn't my back hurt?" "You are having referred pain." "Why does it burn to pee?" "The stone is in the intramural portion of the ureter; it is **at** the bladder and irritating it." "So the stone is in my bladder?" "No, it still has an inch or so to go; it is in the lining of the bladder." "If it is in the bladder then why is the tip of my penis hurting?" And this is why urology is a specialty.*

23
Hematospermia Don't Mean a Thing

Urology Clinic-The Medical College of Georgia

There is an overhead page in the urology clinic. Dr. Gamble, the chief resident, picks up the phone. "There is an internal medicine doctor on the line. He says he has paged you three times today. Can you speak to him?"

Pushing the button for line one an obviously annoyed Dr. Gamble says, "Gamble."

"Oh hi, this is Dr. Gayle. I am one of the internal medicine interns here at Talmadge."

"Yes?"

"We have this patient we would like you to see. He is on our service for a myriad of reasons, but in the course of the work up for diabetes, the nurses have noted blood in his ejaculate. Would you be able to see him today?"

"This happened in the hospital? God!"

"Yes sir. The nurses have paged me several times and they are quite concerned. Blood is everywhere on the sheets. There were even clots!"

Dr. Gamble nonchalantly and in a most condescending tone embellished by a strong southern drawl says, "Hematospermia is a benign process and nothing else need be done at this time. Goodbye."

Slamming the phone down he adds, "These people!"

Rule: Hematospermia is an impressive occurrence and alarming to the patient and nursing staff alike, however, rarely is related to a disease process. In private practice, one would be more tactful in explaining the nuances of this malady. We worry more about blood in the urine than blood at the beginning of the stream, at the end of the stream, blood in the underwear or in the semen.

Urologist to old man: "We need a urine, sperm and stool specimen." The man says to his wife, "What did he say?" She grimaces and says loudly in his ear, "He said to show him your underwear."

24
Beware of Enemy Territory

Enemy territory is that term used when a patient you have operated on shows up at an outlying hospital and is seen by another urologist. You would a colleague in urology, upon seeing a patient of another brother in arms, would manage a patient of yours the way he would want his patient managed by you. *Au contraire!*

I had this forty year or so old patient with refractory testicle pain. On exam, the pain was isolated to the head of the epididymis and very much consistent with chronic epididymitis. He had failed conservative measures, and we agreed to an epididymectomy which I did through a scrotal incision. Beneath the epididymis was a lima bean sized area of firmness consistent with a testis tumor. What to do?

After speaking with a family member, I elected to remove the testicle. I had already made the scrotal incision and I did not see much purpose in removing it through an inguinal approach, so I just took the cord as high as possible. I explained to the patient everything that had happened and what would to expect going forward. He declined arrangements by me for oncological and radiation therapy consultation. He said he was moving to Atlanta, and that he'd get his follow up there. Two years later and on the last day within the statute of limitations, I receive, by way of a Sherriff in my waiting room, a lawsuit. In the papers, there is mention of what a urologist in Atlanta told the patient regarding his treatment by me in the hick town of Gainesville, Georgia.

"The urologist up there must not know what he's doing and he has probably not been well trained. No urologist worth anything would approach a testicle cancer through the scrotum," **Rule: When seeing a patient of another urologist, remember the urologic golden rule: Treat others as you would want to be treated. The jury returned in my favor after forty minutes.**

"The second ideal has been to act the Golden Rule, as far as in me lay, towards my professional brethren and towards the patients committed to my care."-Osler

25

Not All Referring Physicians Are Created Equal

"There are only two sorts of doctors; those who practice with their brains and those who practice with their tongues."-Osler

Fairly early on in my career, I was stopped by an older family medicine doctor and asked if I would review a file for him. I welcomed the opportunity as I was new and my patient load was very light, actually way too light. My wife kept asking me why I was showing up at home so often before lunch, "To work on the swing set," I'd say. Anyway, I go to this doctor's office and he has an entire file that his son, a lawyer, had asked him to review for him.

The case had to do with a percutaneous nephrostolithotomy that had gone bad. You know the drill, the radiologist has trouble obtaining access, and there is bleeding upon dilation of the tract and the case ultimately aborted because lack of visualization secondary to the bleeding: bleeding that required a transfusion, an extended hospital stay, and a discharge with the stone and a nephrostomy in tow.

At the time, I had not been sued yet, so I did not know the nuances of lawsuits and such; but, I did know that not all cases go the way they are planned, and that shit, does indeed, happen.

"Dr. Walker, obviously the details of this case are unfortunate, however, this kind of thing happens often. This type of case either goes very well or it doesn't. If the question is whether this type of thing happens often and does it happen to folks who do this procedure appropriately and often, then the answer is yes," I said.

Dr. Walker told his son what I had said, and the son did not take the case. Dr. Walker then began sending me patients to see in a steady stream until he retired and then became one of my patients. It was in seeing his patients that I learned that a good family doctor has good patients. By that I mean salt of the earth type of patients that are good people and, in turn, are usually compliant with their medicines and grateful for your help. His patients were always a joy to see and so were these patients' family.

My brother Rushton, a musician and a beautiful person, was dying of a base of tongue cancer. I was able to witness many friends of his drop by to pay their respect. They were all so very nice and many brought a guitar along to sing songs they had written for him. I asked him how it was he has so many thoughtful and talented friends. In a raspy voice hard to discern he said, "Culling the dullards."

Rule: Cull the dullards. This requires a conscious effort in terms of your professional life just as it occurs naturally in your personal life. You want "salt of the earth" folks in both realms.

"Save the fleeting minute; learn gracefully to dodge the bore."
-Osler

26
Try to Explain All the Symptoms on the Basis of One Disease

Patients can be funny, and by that I mean odd. When it comes to giving you their history, all the symptoms begin to pile on. You can have a patient with a legitimate problem, but the symptoms that you are given to make a diagnosis go all over the place.

"I get chills and it burns when I urinate. I have a headache in the morning, my lower back hurts, and I stay nauseated all the time."

Now, how in the world do you make sense of all that? Do you think that maybe this patient has stone, meningitis, an ulcer, and is in pending sepsis?

No. Although I have written elsewhere that two diseases can be present at the same time, more often than not there is only one disease. What if the family doctor had given this patient an antibiotic and pyridium for symptoms of a bladder infection, and the pyridium caused the nausea? She stopped drinking coffee and got headaches. The dysuria and lower back is the urinary tract infection, and I don't know what in the hell "chills with voiding means," but I hear that often.

I think the chills with voiding are just an added bonus of the patient trying to explain something that may or may not exist. I remember there was a question we were told to ask the patient who answered in the affirmative every question in the HPI.

"Does your spine itch?" This question works every time; if the answer is yes, then they are either lying or they are crazy.

Rule: It makes more sense that a patient would have only one thing wrong with them, and that this is causing the myriad of symptoms. Remember the patient's personality has a role in the history they give you. Think stoic vs. drama. It can work both ways.

"One swallow does not a summer make, but one tophus makes gout and one crescent, malaria."
-Osler

27
You'll Never Be Faulted for Placing a Stent

What do you think is the most common reason for not placing a stent? It wouldn't be that it is technically difficult to do, or that it has risks that might outweigh the benefits, would it? For me, not placing a stent has a lot to do with worrying about the discomfort of the patient.

Why do something you don't need? Not placing a stent means making some assumptions about the ureter that really one cannot make with accuracy. For instance, an uncomplicated distal stone extraction shouldn't need a stent but on the other hand you have no idea whether there will later be ureteral colic from edema. The patient calling with pain and on his way to the ER will make you rethink your decision. You tried to spare the patient the discomfort and inconvenience of a stent but by doing so made things more difficult for both you and the patient.

In other words, don't over think a stent. If you think about it, then put one in. I never want to be insensitive to the patient who has to endure one. But in the long run, a stent with a string has more positives than negatives.

Years ago, I was asked to see a patient intraoperatively by a gynecologist who was concerned that he may have injured the ureter during a laparoscopic hysterectomy. He had opened the bladder and did not see urine emanating from the left orifice. Upon arriving, I placed a pediatric feeding tube up the ureter without noting any unusual resistance and when I removed it there was prompt efflux of clear urine from the orifice which I observed to continue for 15 minutes of observation. I saw no reason to place a stent particularly since the gynecologist stated that nothing unusual had happened in the course of his surgery.

However, the question had been raised, despite what my evaluation determined, and placing a stent would have been a reasonable action; if for no other reason than providing for a "sleeper stitch "of sorts.

The patient had an unremarkable hospital stay, but represented two weeks later with left ureteral obstruction from a golf ball sized distal urinoma. A different urologist was unable to place a stent, so the patient had a nephrostomy done and then referred to a tertiary care facility to have a ureteral reimplant. The procedure went well, but the patient developed a wound infection which progressed to necrotizing fasciitis, which resulted in a prolonged hospitalization and other surgeries. The gynecologist and I were then sued two years later. After two weeks in court, I was dismissed on summary judgment and the gynecologist was subsequently cleared of mal practice.

Rule: Sometimes a stent protects not just the patient, but also you. A sleeper stitch, a sleeper stent: A stich or stent placed to assure that *you* get a good night's sleep.

"The general who wins battles makes many calculations in his temple before the battle is fought. The general who loses makes but few calculations beforehand."
- Sun Tzu

28
Is Monday Too Soon?

As chief resident in urology, all of the calls about accepting patients from outlying hospitals came to me. And, as usual, the calls most commonly occurred close to five o-clock on a Friday. The reason Friday is the preferred day for a private practice urologist to refer to a teaching institution is because that clears up the problem patient for the weekend. As was made clear to all of the residents, the referrals from private practice urologists, many of whom are alumni of the program, are the lifeblood of the program. The trick then, as is true for me in private practice, is to control the timing of when you accept a patient. One of the reasons most people go into urology is the paucity of emergencies and having to go in at night.

For this reason one of our attendings called urology "gentleman surgery." This refers, of course, to the control we have over when we do our urologic procedures, not to the organ we often have to work on.

Remembering the adage, "It's not what you say but how you say it, and timing is everything." I came upon a response to the five o-clock calls that worked like a charm and I want share it with you now.

"Dr. McHugh, I have a patient in whom I performed a straight forward (they are all straight forward) TURP on and he is requiring around the clock irrigation. My facility is not set up to monitor or treat such a patient. Would your team be of any help to me?"

"Yes sir. We will be very happy to help and accept this patient."

Pause and silence to the point of beginning to feel uncomfortable; and then say: "Would Monday be too soon?"

Rule: When possible, and if medically ethical, help, but on your terms. "Poor planning on their part does not constitute an emergency on yours."

"All men can see these tactics whereby I conquer, but what none can see is the strategy out of which victory is evolved."-Sun Tzu

29
Go Where the Money Is

One of the reasons that I went into urology is that it was something I understood. It was very clear to me that I was not to be a "limp wristed, spine of jelly, lily faced" internal medicine doctor. (That outburst was the line of a fellow urology resident, not my own.)

I loved all the sayings, aphorisms, maxims and adages that each of the older residents and attendings would pass on. Most were mentioned in passing and used to complement a teaching point and did facilitate learning. I loved them and none more than the one regarding Willie Sutton, the 1920's American bank robber.

The story goes that when asked why he robbed banks, he replied, "That's where the money is." As it turns out, he was interviewed after being paroled in the 1960's and said that he had not made that statement, although he felt the conclusion was obvious.

Now known as Sutton's Law, the concept is to order tests keeping in mind that diagnosis which would be most likely to be present; in other words "when you hear hoof beats, think horses not zebras" and act accordingly.

Sutton stole over 2 million dollars, never killed anyone (you can't say that about doctors), used an unloaded gun, and stated: "I never felt so much alive as when I robbed banks."

Rule: If the patient has pain at McBurney's Point, then don't go looking in the ears.

"Move not unless you see an advantage; use not your troops unless there is something to be gained; fight not unless the position is critical."-Sun Tzu

30
When All Else Fails Blame the Patient

The patient is a valuable resource when it comes to surgical outcomes that just don't turn out right. Some surgeons use this resource more commonly than others. You know who I'm talking about, I bet.

One way to assure that the patient is to blame for any problem with surgery is to give hard to follow post-operative instructions. I personally don't use a certain amount of weight as an instruction but many physicians do. What exactly is fifteen pounds? I know that is not much, certainly less than picking up a baby. So a lady has a C-section and is strategically told not to lift more than fifteen pounds for six weeks. The likelihood is that she is doomed to fail in accomplishing this restriction.

When she shows up with a small dehiscence of the incision or say soreness of the incision, the physician then can dutifully ask, "Have you lifted anything over fifteen pounds?" The answer is most likely yes and there you have it. It wasn't the surgery. It was the patient not following very clear and implicit instructions.

Here's another favorite of mine that I have heard on many occasions. Let's say that I am planning to do a scrotal hydrocelectomy on a patient, and in the process of the explanation the patient has a question.

"I need to tell you something. The last surgery I had for a hernia it took six weeks for me to heal. It opened up real bad because my body rejected the suture. The doctor said I was probably allergic to it. If something bad is going to happen to someone it will be me."

Don't snatch defeat from the jaws of victory. If the patient wants to take the blame for something untoward about your surgery, who are you to stop him?

Rule: Oh no, it couldn't be the surgeon's fault, his technique or an infection could it? The patient's body "rejected it."
If the patient tells you that, "If something bad is going to happen to someone it will happen to me," don't dissuade him from it...that's your back up scape goat.

31

Two Different Diseases Can Occur at the Same Time

Well, you have to at least think about it; two processes going on at the same time. I know I have another aphorism about trying to explain all the symptoms on the basis of one disease, but this is the reverse corollary.

Here's one that will get you. The patient has a known history of kidney stones and has right flank pain and hematuria. All of the associated stone symptoms are present and the radiation of pain fits the diagnosis of colic. In this patient, however, there is a touch of nausea and some of the pain radiates to the middle of the back.

This patient's pain is such that she requires admission for intractable pain and the CT scheduled. The CT shows stones in the kidney but no ureteral stones. There is mild fullness of the right renal pelvis but no associated caliectasis. So, the fullness throws you a bit. Maybe there is a passed stone but there is no perinephric stranding. Okay, no stones in the gallbladder per the CT. There is one problem; the patient is still in pain and requiring parenteral analgesics. She is reliable and not a pain seeker. Hmmmmmmmmm.

On a whim, a DISIDA scan is ordered and voilà, there is a functional obstruction of the gallbladder, which is subsequently removed and the now the patient is all better.

Rule: "A patient can have lice and fleas at the same time."-Osler.

Corollary: Patients tend to temporally, and conveniently I might add, relate a problem to the time of a procedure you performed on them. Example: "Ever since the vasectomy my sex drive is nonexistent. Also the head of my penis has no sensitivity since you did the vasectomy. You could drag it over sand paper and I wouldn't feel it. Is it possible you messed something up in there? I had none of these symptoms before you worked on me."

32
Treatment Plan? Which Month is It?

"When I was a boy of fourteen, my father was so ignorant I could hardly stand to have the old man around. But when I got to be twenty-one, I was astonished at how much the old man had learned in seven years."-Twain

S ometimes what is frustrating can, if managed appropriately, work to one's advantage. In my residency program, like others I am sure, we had several attendings and each had his own way of "doing business." Some were prone to surgical solutions for a particular problem, others much more conservative in pursuing operative intervention. Each was given certain months to be the rounding attending, so you knew well in advance who you'd have to run a case by. In other words, if you had a patient with an invasive bladder tumor and hoping to do a cystectomy, your chances of getting to do the case were better on a month with a surgical minded attending. This is not a statement as to one philosophy being right or wrong or better than the other; just how it was.

The frustration part of this arrangement manifested itself in having to not only figure out what treatment plan was correct but to do so with the mindset of the attending *du jour*. In a way, the complexity of this circuitous route to treatment was in itself an education; in retrospect it made the program better. There are indeed, more than ways than one to skin the cat.

So, over time I learned to use our attending situation as a teachable moment whenever a junior resident presented a case to me.

Regarding a potential cystectomy patient and asked if a particular patient would be a candidate I would reply," Well that depends."

"What do you mean, that depends?" would be the response.

"Well," I'd say, "it depends on what month it is."

"It is April, what does that have to with it?"

"Well, if it is April, then that means this patient needs a bone scan, an updated cystoscopy, a radiation consult, an oncology consult, medical clearance, confirmation of muscle invasion by your personal review of the pathology slides with the pathologist, ostomy clinic evaluation of where the stoma will be and that the body habitus is suitable for the collection appliance, a thorough discussion with the patient and family of the risks as well as all other options for therapy to include doing nothing, and then, once that is done, presenting the case to the attending of the month of April."

"On the other hand," I continued. "If the month is May, then get all your ducks in a row, and we'll present the case to the attending and hopefully put the patient on for the first available day on the operative schedule."

Rule: You have your whole career to do things your way. As a resident, don't fight the advice or methods of the attendings; glean everything you can from them and assimilate that into your clinical armamentarium when for you're in charge. What I thought at the time was a weakness of our program was actually the strength of it. The obvious is sometimes difficult to discern, especially to the myopic young. Do as I say not as I have done.

It takes a wise man to learn from his mistakes; even a wiser man to learn from others.

"Common-sense nerve fibers are seldom medullated before forty-they are never seen even with a microscope before twenty."- Osler

Youth is wasted on the young...so too is advice.

The next time a junior resident asks you how to get a particular case by a particular attending, do your hands like Mr. Miyagi in the movie, "The Karate Kid" and say in a Chinese accent the words of Sun Tzu:

"Grasshopper, water shapes its course according to the nature of the ground over which it flows; the soldier works out his victory in relation to the foe whom he is facing. Therefore, just as water retains no constant shape, so in warfare there are no constant conditions. He who can modify his tactics in relation to his opponent and thereby succeed in winning, may be called a heaven-born captain. Now...wax on-wax off."

33
Prostates Have to Vine Ripen

Have you ever noticed how neurosurgeons handle the patient with chronic back pain? Those patients are told to wait to have anything surgically done until the pain is unbearable. In other words, they are told to elect to have surgery as the last resort. In many ways this is not a bad surgical philosophy for any malady for which there is a surgical option. This technique is protective as it assures that the patient has been given conservative options and there has been no rush to surgery. If there is less than optimal outcome, then the surgeon will less likely be blamed. This is a corollary of the "when all else fails, blame the patient."

"Yes sir, I am sorry that your back pain is not completely resolved. That is why I was hesitant to pursue surgery, but as we discussed, we were out of options. So, now, what about that pesky prostate and when should you operate?"

In the case of the enlarged prostate and its attendant obstructive voiding symptoms, one does not want to intervene too soon. The more dramatic the preoperative obstructive voiding symptoms, the more dramatic improvement will be perceived by the patient. That is what you want to achieve. Suggesting the possibility of the patient's diet having a role, trying all the medicines available for prostatism, and preoperative cystoscopic evaluation to get the lay of the land are all key elements in setting the stage for the urologist suggesting intervention. More importantly, the patient will feel all the conservative measures have been tried and be more willing to advance to the next step.

Rule: Remember you can almost assure that the stream will be better (obstructive symptoms); however, you cannot assure that there will be less frequency or nocturia (irritative symptoms). You wouldn't pick a tomato too soon would you?

"I watched what method Nature might take, with intention of subduing the symptom by treading in her footsteps."-Sydenham

34

A Man Spends His First Fifty Years Making a Living-The Second Fifty Trying to Make Water

The saying about boiling crabs and frogs comes to mind. It is something about if the water is heated slowly to a boil they won't fight it and will be cooked peacefully. So too is the indolent presentation of obstructive voiding symptoms. Now don't get me wrong; the patient will swear that the prostate symptoms came on all of a sudden.

In reality, however, the symptoms came on very gradually and unnoticed by the patient until he has to get up at night.

To the patient with a very large post void residual noted on bladder ultrasound you ask, "Do you have any trouble making your water?"

"None at all, I go all the time," is the reply. (Overflow incontinence)

On further questioning you elicit the history of sitting to void, hesitancy, nocturia, stop-start stream, stranguria and the like; but slow stream often times is not the complaint.

I examined a patient once whose bladder was to the umbilicus (even I could tell that wasn't normal) and then asked if he had any problem peeing.

"Not at all," was the reply despite a basketball sized bladder.

So, what do you do if you have trouble getting the obstructive history? Try asking these visually intensive questions:

- Can you write your name in the snow?
- Can you knock the bark of a tree?
- Can you knock gravel over in the parking lot?
- Can you pee and run under it?
- Do men come and go in the bathroom before you finish?
- Can you pee like a race horse?

- Can you pee over a fence post?

With these answers in hand and with a smile on the face of the patient for having asked in this way, you are well on your way to the determining the severity of the voiding issues.

Rule: Men are poor historians when it comes to an accurate history of their voiding symptoms. Although they will speak of the irritative symptoms freely, chief among them nocturia, obstruction by the prostate is usually the culprit. You have to make very clear to the patient that the procedure recommended to open the prostate is to make the flow better and hopefully improve the nocturia. Otherwise the patient comes back after the surgery saying, "The procedure did not work. I can pee like a water faucet but I still get up at night."

"If a patient does not remember the making of his water, then he is in a dangerous situation."-Hippocrates

35
Keep Your Nose Clean

I am from LaGrange, Georgia, and grew up one block off the square in my grandmother's house: the house in which my mother grew up. Sitting on the front porch and watching people go to the Presbyterian Church, which was across the street, or commenting on those going to shop at Mansour's were our favorite pastime. It was on that porch that I envisioned "making a doctor," working as a physician down the street at a clinic named for a good friend of my grandfather, and walking to my grandmother's house for lunch every day.

The urologists in LaGrange had intimated an interest in my joining their group and had indicated there might be a spot with them when I had finished the last year of my residency. As it turned out, they hired someone who was immediately available and my opportunity with them, the only group of urologists in LaGrange, vanished. I still wanted to live in LaGrange; my wife was a bit less sure as my mother was a bit "too much." There was a group of physicians not associated with the clinic who were looking to start another urology group. They called me and I went to interview and meet those doctors. During the course of my visit, I bumped into one of the urologists in the group that had chosen another urologist.

After subtleties, the urologist said, "John, you know that if you come here, we will not cover call with you and if you get in trouble in the operating room we can't guarantee that we'd be there to help you."

As a junior resident, the thought of not having back up and taking call every day was intimidating. Whatever the guy had hoped to achieve was successful. I decided to look elsewhere, which suited my wife just fine. I mentioned what had happened to Dr. Witherington in Augusta, and he said, "John, if you want to go to LaGrange, go and keep your nose clean. In time, there will be a day that they need you to take call for them, and when you do everything will be all right."

Rule: A competing urology group, in time, will need your help.

36

Do You See That Big Silver Building Over There?

I was an intern on a general surgery service at University Hospital in Augusta, Georgia. The teaching hospital, Talmadge Memorial, was across the street from the new VA hospital and just a few blocks from University Hospital. The three formed a triangle. You could see each of the other hospitals from any one of the three. The VA hospital was sliver; it looked a lot like how stainless steel kitchen appliances look. It stood out compared to the older hospitals constructed of traditional brick and mortar. This was highlighted by the way it reflected sunlight.

One morning on rounds at University Hospital, an intern began to give the history of an unfortunate soul who had been admitted after having been found unconscious under a bridge. She began to give the history to include his admission vital signs, her exam, and the litany of blood work she had obtained. Nothing she mentioned indicated that the patient had anything that needed surgery and as such, the chief surgical resident did not seem overly interested in the presentation. Well, that was until she mentioned where the patient had had an appendectomy during the Second World War.

"This patient had surgery in the forties when he was stationed in Kansas," she said.

The chief resident perked up, "Stationed in Kansas? He served in the military?"

"Yes sir."

The chief resident, as he is pulling the curtain back behind the patient's bed to reveal the sun drenched VA hospital, says, "Dr. Smith, do you see that silver building over there? Please have this patient in that building before rounds tomorrow morning. Is that clear?"

Rule: The history of the patient is very important. You have to keep your service clean.

37
Do You Think this is Wal-Mart or Something?

There are a lot of brash and know-it-all doctors out there that are all full of themselves. You know the type I'm talking about. However true this may be, these peacocks of the medical profession are, at times, interesting to observe. To some extent, this type of character may have been more prevalent in the earlier days of medicine than presently.

One such man that comes to mind was the senior partner of the oldest internal medicine group in our city. I met him when I first came to town and was going around introducing myself to all the doctors. That's right. All new doctors to town used to do that! I wait to see this guy, and when I finally get to see him he says to me, "You need to tell your partner to shut up! You don't get to be the lead dog just because you talk a lot. He needs to go to the back of the pack." Apparently, my new partner was unpopular with this doctor; so much for referrals from this giant of the community.

The story goes that this doctor was walking into the emergency room when a patient lying on a stretcher in the hall yelled out and pointed in his direction.

Waking up from an apparent stupor the patient says, "I'll take that one."

When the doctor realized that the patient was referring to him he replied as he neared the stretcher.

"This ain't Wal-Mart!" he replied and kept on walking. It was a great line and now is part of urban legend in my town.

Rule: Just because something is inappropriate doesn't mean that it isn't true.

"Acquire the art of detachment, the virtue of method, the quality of thoroughness, but above all else the grace of humility."-Osler

38
You and God Weren't Doing So Well Before I Got Here

An old-school cardiologist had been called to intensive care one evening to see a patient in congestive heart failure who was going south. Throughout the evening and into the next morning, he used all of his tricks to stabilize the rhythm and diuresis the fluid from the patient's lungs. This resulted in a remarkable turnaround, and, as the sun was rising and the light began filtering into the room, several family members entered. The doctor began to give an update as to the patient's condition and at the tail end of this the preacher arrived. When the doctor had finished and began to leave the room, the preacher attempted to stop him.

"May we have a word of prayer?" the preacher asked, much to the chagrin of the tired physician who had been at the patient's bedside all night.

The preacher continued, "May we all bow our heads and hold hands? I want to thank the good Lord for getting our brother Bill through such a perilous evening and give thanks for his miraculous improvement this morning."

The physician did not heed the attempt to stop his departure nor the preacher's request for prayer.

"You and God weren't doing so well before I got here!" he said and walked out of the intensive care area.

Rule: God heals the patient and the doctor renders the bill; and don't you forget it. A word to the wise is sufficient.

"Prayer indeed is good, but while calling on the gods the man himself should lend a hand."-Hippocrates

"Knowing not whence he came, why he is here, or whither he is going, man feels himself of supreme importance, and certainly of interest-to himself. Let us hope that he has indeed a potency and importance out of all proportion to his somatic insignificance." -Osler

39

Deliberate 24 Hours before Agreeing to Switch Call

I have a brother who is in sales. He is good at it and loves the dynamics of making a sell. The very thing that you or I would hate about selling things to people, he loves and embraces. "You gotta get to no, John. You gotta have an objection. Without an objection, you will never understand the buyer and if you don't understand the buyer's concerns, how will you never sell him on the benefits of your product?"

He gave me all these Zig Zigler cassette tapes years ago and I was fascinated by them. He's good, he made his fame in selling pots and pans and then later as a motivational speaker and writer. What's nice about knowing the above is that it helps you when sales people use their techniques on you. Once, a traveling meat salesman showed up at my door. You know the kind with the small truck with a refrigerated compartment in the back. "I am not interested," I say.

"You are not interested in saving money?" he replies.

Here's the thing. You cannot give them any information to build on or base the next question on. Do not give them an objection-they have a ready response to that. Trust me.

"I am not interested in saving money," I say.

"You are telling me that you want to have to drive to a store to buy steaks and pay more for it?" he says as I am inching the door shut.

"Yes," I say. I knew the drill. "Goodbye," I say.

The same rationale applies to swapping call. The person requesting the change knows the weekend he wants off is the day of the big game, the big game party, and E.R. call. He asks you on the fly; most likely while in the midst of doing some task that favors you answering quickly and in the affirmative.

Rule: Resist the urge to change anything until you have had 24 hours to look at a calendar and speak to your wife. The salesman and that guy who is always switching the call schedule are in the know, and have the advantage from the get go.

40
Have You Ever Sewn in a Drain Dr. Dixon?

P.K. Dixon was one of the first general surgeons in our area. He was in his seventies and actively practicing when I came to Gainesville. He was a man's man of sorts, an excellent surgeon and a strong-willed individual, as well.

I had done a partial nephrectomy on a child for a supernumerary kidney, and a day later, when I went to remove the drain, it would not come out. I had sewn it to the fascia deep within the flank.

"I'll be back later in the day to work on this," I say to the family not really knowing what I was going to do.

I see Dr. Dixon in the surgical changing room and decide to get his thoughts on my dilemma. I felt very bad about this. Because of my error, I may be subjecting this child and family to an additional procedure, pain, and risk.

"Dr. Dixon, I did a nephrectomy on a child yesterday, and when I attempted to remove the penrose it would not come out. I think I have sewn it in at the level of the fascia. Has that ever happened to you?" I ask.

He is pulling on his scrub pants and looks at me over the rims of his bifocals. After a pause and cinching the scrubs tight, he says with a grin, "Maybe two or three... hundred times."

Confident people can be brutally honest. How can you argue or find fault or judge someone who is honest? You can't. You can tell who is honest and who is a white lie type of person. People who are fudging use way too many words. Twain said, "If you tell the truth you don't have to remember anything."

Rule: You admire more the doctors who are honest than the ones that let on that nothing bad ever happens in their hands. If you play golf with a doctor that cheats, then don't send him patients.

"If you ain't wrecking, you ain't racing."-Richard Petty

If a surgeon tells you that "in my hands" he has not had this or that complication doing a certain procedure then he hasn't done enough of that procedure.

41
You Shudda Drinned Him

Ken Dixon, the son of P.K. Dixon and a general surgeon, as well, has shared many stories related to him by his dad. My favorite had to do with one of the first surgeons in our area and the undertaker.

The undertaker was fond of second guessing the cause of death and medical management of those unfortunate souls who ended up needing his services. On one occasion, the mortician was speaking to the family of a patient who had just died of appendicitis.

"Your father probably would not have died if he'd had a drin. The doctor shudda drinned him," he says.

About a month later, another patient has passed away from appendicitis and again the undertaker was consoling the family.

"You mother would not have died had the doctor not placed a drin. He shuddna drinned him."

The surgeon of the two victims of appendicitis heard tell of the undertaker's Monday morning quarterbacking and decided to pay him a visit. This surgeon was known to keep a pearl handled revolver in his bedside table. He made a point to take the gun with him for his trip to the funeral home.

The surgeon finds the funeral director sitting at his desk and approaches him with the gun pointed at his head.

"If I hear about you telling a family again that I should have or should not have placed a drain, I am going to drin you six times!"

Rule: Bart Simpson was placed in a gifted class at school by accident. He was asked his opinion as to why some countries rationalize the ambivalent argument that spending money on a strong defense is actually a deterrent to war. He said, "Well, I guess you are damned if you do and damned if you don't." Sometimes in medicine you are damned if you do and damned if you don't.

You don't always have the benefit of the "retrospective scope." It seems, however, that everyone else does.

42
Look at What They Are Looking At

I love history. And of all the historical figures I have read about, none interests me more than Will Rogers. No, no, not Roy and not Buck, but Will Rogers of Oklahoma. In the 1920s and 1930s he was the highest paid and most beloved entertainer in America. He was one-fourth Cherokee, and began his career by doing tricks with ropes. The story goes that he got his big break during a performance in New York in which he messed up the rope trick and said, "I guess I can't throw a rope and chew gum at the same time." He then walked to the wings of the stage and stuck his gum on the wall and continued the performance. The crowd responded so enthusiastically that he then did the mistake and the remark on purpose for each successive show. In time he added more dialogue which then resulted in a show primarily discussing the news in a clever and funny way.

"All I know is what I've read in the paper," he'd say. One of his famous quotes, and there are hundreds, was, " If you want to know why a man acts the way he does, walk around behind him and look out at what he is looking at."

This saying works well when dealing with difficult patients or, more commonly, their family. The patient is sick; he is scared and doesn't feel well. The family, for reasons we always don't understand, over-dramatize their love for the patient, and, in turn, they feel they have to be demanding and protect their loved one. Many have not been ideal children and have chosen the current situation to show their love, but in an inappropriate manor. We get what's going on; it is a time of stress and people act differently. I say look at what they are looking at and give them a pass. You have to recognize what is happening and why, and then you can hopefully act with compassion.

Rule: Someone asked Will Rogers how it was he could get away with making fun of Presidents and then be invited back the next year to do the same thing again. He said, "They are big people."

Let us strive to be big doctors.

43
What Would You Do If You Were Me?

This question, by the patient of the doctor who has rightfully given and explained all of the options to manage the issue at hand, is a common and appropriate question to ask.

The problem, however, is that the doctor is not the patient.

"I am not you. You and I are different, are of a different age, and have different factors in our lives that will affect the decision process."

Now, the doctor does not have to say that but the above response is the essence of answering the question. In the book I wrote, *The Decision*, I take pains to outline a decision worksheet that takes in account all of the factors in the decision making process if you have prostate cancer.

"I can answer that question if you tell me a little about yourself," is the right answer. This question will allow you to know the patient better and help both you and he arrive at the decision best for *him*.

"I don't want any chance of impotence or incontinence," the patient says. Well, if I were him, then I'd choose radiation. "I don't care about potential impotence or incontinence; I want the most aggressive option with the best chance of cure." Well, if I am that patient, then I'd pursue a prostatectomy.

Rule: In advising the patient regarding treatment, sometimes what to do is more about what is best for the patient and not what is best for the disease.

"The good physician treats the disease; the great physician treats the patient who has the disease."-Osler

44
Always Have a Toy Box

There's the cutest little patient of mine who is in his eighties. When he comes to the office, he always brings me something. Usually the gift is from Jaemor Farms, a local country store surrounded by a fruit orchard. Usually the gift is either peaches, if they are in season, or a specialty bread they make using the fruit they grow. He told me that when he was growing up his father was a gift giver.

"No one ever came to our house without leaving with something. My father made sure that everybody got something. I am the same way. I got it from my father."

This brings me to the toy box. You got to have a toy box in the office. For forty dollars you get about a hundred simple toys that are an absolute joy to give out to children. But here's the secret. Older patients love the toys too. It is not the toy alone, but the giving that invariably makes a person smile. How about a little soldier with a parachute, or a little hand clapper, kazoo or those gooey figures that stick to the wall when you throw them?

Recently, the toy box came with a Chinese finger trap. This is a particularly fun way to play with children but also is an excellent tool to show how the tension free sling works. It's a perfect teaching aid.

No child? No problem. You give a toy to the patient to give a child or grandchild.

If I have seen it once, I have seen it a thousand times; a child running to the toy box and then kneeling in front of it to go through the toys to pick something out. There is always a thank you from the parent, as well.

"You can only have five," I usually tell them.

Rule: Make your office fun if you can. Adding a toy box will help. Can you make animal balloons? I can. It's easy!

The dour physician is repulsive to the well and sick alike.

45
When All Else Fails Ask the Patient

A patient is lying in his bed surrounded by several members of the urology service rounding team. Let's see, there is the attending, the chief resident, a junior resident, an intern or two, several students and a nurse. The patient is listening while the team talks about him. This is one of the hard things to get used to in a teaching hospital; talking about the patient's medical problems in front of him. In time, it becomes second nature to both the training doctor and the patient.

On one occasion, the attending asks the chief resident if the patient had had his IVP that morning. The chief resident looks to the junior resident who looks at an intern who looks to the students. The students think to look at the nurse, but think better of it.

The intern queries the students, "Did Mr. Smith have the IVP this morning?"

The two students then look at each other. And the looking at each other continues up the line in an opposite direction back to the attending. Then everybody just looks at each other.

The patient says, "I had it this morning about seven. The radiologist told me it was normal."

Rule: The diagnosis can be determined 85% of the time from the history gleaned from the patient. Corollary: 15% of the patients have 85% of the diseases.

God gave you two ears and one mouth for a reason.

46

The Scrotum is Your Friend-The Urethra is Your Enemy

One of the few presentations I made as a resident to the Southeast Section of the American Urologic association was on Fournier's gangrene. Our teaching hospital had a rash of this disease, and it prompted the head of the department to have me choose this as a topic. It is a fairly simple disease, essentially a necrotizing fasciitis with its origin in or about the scrotum. I had the original article in French by Fournier and had it translated for my paper at the tune of $375.00, much to the chagrin of the attendings. I thought they had given me permission for the expense.

Two things about this disease and the treatment of it; the testicles are spared because they have a different unaffected blood supply, and you can remove almost all the scrotum and it will find a way to cover the testicles, in time.

"John, you only need a postage stamp of a scrotum to cover the testicles," Dr. Witherington would tell me.

Now take a look at that sorry assed and vindictive urethra; absolutely no forgiveness and nothing but prolonged anguish. You think you can cure a stricture? The urethra laughs at you. You use the urethra to get to the prostate and damage it. You think it forgets? Hell no! If it had a motto it would be "Don't tread on me."

There was a patient who had pan urethral stricture disease in whom we perpetrated upon him one of those English procedures where you open up the entire length of the penis and urethra with the plan to make a new urethra several months later; an overcooked Ballpark frank comes to mind.

On rounds, a resident seeing the result for the first time said to the patient, "You let a doctor do that to you?"

Rule: The urethra doesn't like being messed with. Tread softly and carefully. There is no fury like a urethra scorned. The scrotum: a loveable fuzz ball.
"In the drama that is Fournier's, the scrotum will give its life for the sake of the testicles."
-McHugh

47
Beware of the Overly Complimentary Patient

S o, you know the story about the guy that shot John Lennon? I might mention that I am a huge Beatles fan. In medical school, I produced a musical opera of sorts to "A Day in the Life" for our freshman class talent show. The next year, I was elected class president. This was probably due to the exposure I got from this skit. Several classmates said I had missed my calling. It was good. I have a picture of me dancing to "When I'm Sixty-Four" with a friend. I changed the words around to state, "I'll probably still be in medical school...when I'm sixty-four."

The guy who shot Lennon loved him. Remember he had read J.D. Salinger's book *Catcher in the Rye*. The guy went to high school in Atlanta, became disenchanted with Lennon, stalked him, and the rest is history. How do you go from admiration to assassination? I think about this when I look at the picture of my children walking across the street to The Dakota, where Lennon was shot, done like the cover of the Abbey Road album.

So too, are the patients that think you hung the moon. Beware of them. The higher they put you on a pedestal, the longer and harder the fall when, for whatever reason, you disappoint them. It might be the bill, having to wait, having to see the nurse practitioner on a busy day, or an interaction with the urologist on call that sets them off. And, they don't just leave; they make a scene out of their departure. A letter, an email, voice messages or calling the administrative staff is done to make sure their grievance is noted by all.

So when a patient says that you come highly regarded and that you are the best urologist in town, be careful.

Rule: With praise comes higher expectations and a greater likelihood of not meeting those expectations. Every happy patient tells one person, but the unhappy patient tells ten.

"They love without measure those whom they will soon hate without reason."
-Sydenham

48
You Are Not That Great a Doctor John, I Trained Him for You

When you have been in practice a while you become less tolerant of inappropriate patients. Although all of us, as a rule, bend over backwards to please patients, sometimes enough is enough and they need to be fired. Just as with children, you cannot continue to reward bad behavior.

When I first moved to Gainesville, there was a nice enough older urologist who had a crusty side. He was in a competing group, but his relationship to me was much like that of a mentor. He stopped me one day coming out of the hospital.

"John, you will probably be seeing a patient of mine for a vasectomy in the near future. He was in the office the other day and was rude to my staff because of having to wait. His name is Jerry Wade and I personally confronted him in our waiting room and told him that I would not be doing his vasectomy and to leave my office. After some harsh words on both of our parts, he left."

"He will probably be coming to you to have the vasectomy done. You will think that he is very nice and courteous and you'll wonder why I had such a problem. You'll probably think that I am the rude one and that I have no bedside manors. You'll also surmise that because of your skills and personality, the patient behaved nicely."

He continued, "Nothing could be further from the truth. He is indeed an inappropriate person and patient. I have trained him for you, he'll be polite for you, and you are welcome."

Rule: I did see the patient and he was delightful. The other urologist trained him quite well. I considered having all my vasectomy pre-ops being screened by this urologist going forward.

"With our History, Tradition, Achievements, and Hopes, there is little room for Chauvinism in medicine."-Osler

49

If It Was Hard for the Urologist before You It Will Be Hard for You Too

I live in Gainesville, Georgia, and I am geographically right between the mountains of Northeast Georgia and Atlanta. To the urologists north of me I am the next line of defense and to whom they would send problem patients to. In turn, Atlanta is where I would send a difficult patient and hence, I become the outlying urologist. As a doctor, you don't mean to, but because you are in a bigger city, or associated with a bigger hospital, you tend to think you might be better at something than that guy in the smaller area. You might even have the ego to think that you are better than any other urologist. So when you get the call, you automatically think that the problems the referring urologist is explaining to you to justify the referral, will not be a problem for you. It is a natural response; resist it.

Think of Shakespeare: "Tis best to weigh the enemy more mighty than he seems."

You think that the urologist in a small hospital up in the mountains who had a problem getting past a small stone in the proximal ureter of pregnant woman will be a breeze for you? Will you attempt to repeat the same procedure he did because *you* can do it? Or will you receive the patient and manage her much as if you had had the problems he experienced? May I suggest the latter?

Truth be known, these guys elsewhere are having to use their skills in urology often times without the back up of an interventional radiologist or all the extra stuff that comes from working in a bigger hospital. I have the utmost respect for them. Let me add, however, I don't want them sending me stuff all the time that they started; that is another matter.

Rule: If someone was operated on by another urologist and it did not go well for him, it will be hard for you. And, always weigh that problem more mighty than it seems. You ain't that special.
"The daily round of a busy practitioner tends to develop an egotism of a most intense kind, to which there is no antidote"-Osler

50

I Am Allergic To Tordol and Ultram-What Are You Going to Give Me?

When a patient with stone pain or one with back pain and a history of stone disease asks what you are going give them for pain, it tells you something. When they add on the allergies to the medicines you'd rather give, then too, you realize this ain't their first rodeo.

I am not saying they are bad people or drug seekers, I am saying they represent a segment of your practice that is a difficult management problem.

If they don't have an obvious stone on KUB but the pain seems legitimate, then you are faced with repeating a CT that they probably have had in the last few months, or giving them pain medicine based on the history.

Here's the thing. If you give pain medicine when you think you probably shouldn't, then you are only perpetuating the problem. In time, you'll learn if this patient is working you or not. When the medicine is used up, this begets another phone call or office visit. When they don't get what they want, they often become belligerent. There will be numerous voice messages, conversations back and forth with your nurses, pain medicines given but the appointment not kept, and ultimately more pain medicine prescribed with the anticipation of ureteroscopy that is, at the last minute, cancelled. I have seen this scenario more times than I can remember.

The solution? I don't have one. I'd say that as soon as this type of stone patient is recognized that he or she be nipped in the bud. Remember Barney Fife on "Andy of Mayberry?" "You gotta nip it Andy. Nip it in the bud!"

Rule: Recognizing something for what it is is the first step.

"One of the first duties of the physician is to educate the masses not to take medicine."-Osler

51

Having Read Something in a Book Don't Mean Jack!

I can remember standing outside of a patient's room with the attending and several residents and interns of the rounding team. It would have been about six at night, toward the end of the day. The patient had an invasive bladder cancer, and we were discussing the management options. Now to set the stage, the attending on this day was of a conservative nature, and that flavored the options and tone of the discussion. The issue was whether pre-cystectomy adjunctive radiation would be done or not. The attending stated that, in this patient, we would arrange for the radiation and the cystectomy would be done after that. Now you have to be in the mind of the resident who wanted to be a part of doing the cystectomy. The radiation meant a delay of weeks, which in turn meant to him that he would be off the Talmadge service and on the V.A. service. So a case that he diagnosed, worked-up, and prepared for the paragon of urologic surgeries would be served on a silver platter to another resident coming onto the service.

"I read in Campbell's that the survival rate with or without radiation is similar and that there are fewer surgical complications without radiation. Can we consider proceeding with cystectomy without the radiation?" the resident asks. The attending's comeback to this particular resident was quite good. Imagine the intonation of the response with a thick northern accent; that makes it all the better.

With hands heavenward and in dramatic fashion the attending looks at the resident and says, "Look everyone, Jerry says he's read something in a book. Wow! He read something in a book and of course that makes it so. Doesn't it Jerry? Jerry is so smart he can read!"

Rule: Take experience over what is written in a book any day.

"He who studies medicine without books sails an uncharted sea, but he who studies medicine without patients does not go to sea at all."-Osler

52

Stand Up and Turn Around in a Circle and Place Hand on Door Knob

I mentioned elsewhere in this book an older family practice doctor who supported me early in my career. His office was near the doctor's parking lot, and often I would walk into the hospital with him. Just as with other physicians I walked into the hospital with from the parking lot, I always learned things from Dr. Walker.

The discussion came up about how to get out of a room of a time-usurping patient when you were behind in the office and had more urgent patients to see. As you know, you don't want to be rude and cut people off, but many times the history you need has been gleaned, and it is time to move on.

Dr. Walker says, "John, I have method that works every time. It is tailor made for that type of patient you can't get out of the room and when the interview has gone on way too long. What you do is to stand up in mid conversation and turn in a complete circle, place a hand on the door knob, and then look over your shoulder back at the patient."

He continued, "You then ask if there are any more questions as you are opening the door. This maneuver has the effect of stunning the patient. They forget where they were in the discourse and will stand up to follow you out. You disclose your treatment on the way to check-out. Works like a charm."

I add that the best time to ask, "Do you have any more questions?" in urology is just after you have done the rectal exam and have handed the patient tissue. Much like standing up and turning around, this urological technique is a diversionary tactic. You ask the question at a time when the patient is preoccupied. This discourages any more questions allows you to leave the room under the guise of giving the patient privacy.

Rule: When patients begin to ask another question before you have answered the first, then it is time to move from history (his turn to talk) to treatment (your turn to talk).

"A patient with a written list of symptoms-neurasthenia."-Osler

53
A Fool with a Tool Is Still a Fool

The percutaneous nephrostolithotomy procedure was in its infancy when I was a resident. So too, the introduction of the interventional radiologist into the lives of the urologic resident was also a new twist. What I remember about this era was that all of the residents wanted to learn to do the placement of the nephrostomy. We couldn't understand at the time why we were beholden to someone else, particularly a radiologist, to be the gate keeper for a disease that was clearly in our bailiwick. From some reason, the residents at Talmadge would do the PNLs at the VA hospital; it may have been they had a newer radiology suite. We'd get there by walking through a long walk way that went over the street between the two hospitals.

The interventional radiologist was quite the character, and, to my knowledge, he was the only one of record for Talmadge, the VA and the private hospital, University Hospital. There may have been others, but he is the only one I remember.

The percutaneous approach and all the instruments used were new to me. This interventional radiologist had every sort of wire, dilators, and access catheters of every description. He was a spectacle to watch and bordered on being theatrical with all the fluid motion of things going in and then coming out; all witnessed by all of us because of fluoroscopy.

Anyway, the thing I remember the most about him is a phrase he would say repeatedly as he demonstrated the process of placing a nephrostomy.

"A fool with a tool is still a fool," he'd say.

Rule: The Da Vinci robot and urologists use of it comes to mind.

"It is astonishing with how little reading a doctor can practice medicine, but it is not astonishing how badly he may do it."-Osler

Like an archer who wounds at random, is he who hires a fool or any passer-by. As a dog returns to its vomit, so a fool repeats his folly. - Proverbs 26:10-11.

54

I Am Not Sure I Understand Everything I Know About This Patient

D o you feel uncomfortable, or have trouble saying (if you ever do), "I don't know?" You really should try it; this response as a physician to a patient's or colleague's question is liberating. Also, it will be viewed as you having experience and wisdom. The admission of not knowing elevates the complexity of the question and gives it more credence.

Now you may not have the confidence to just say, "I don't know." I understand. You may not have that level of maturity yet; you have not come full circle in knowledge. Knowing you don't know is wisdom.

Well, if you are like many and you can't stand not appearing knowledgeable, then let me offer a compromise phrase to you. This was used by an older vascular surgeon in response to questions about a train wreck of a patient and what exactly was to be done with him.

Wait for it. First, remember what Churchill said about negotiating with Russia:

"It is a riddle wrapped in a mystery inside an enigma; but perhaps there is a key."

Some patients, their medical conditions, and the management or the order of the management often exemplify this quote.

So, what did the attending say to the difficult question posed by the chief vascular resident?

"I am not sure that I understand all I know about this patient."

Not quite Churchill but pretty darn good I thought.

Rule: Don't feel like you always have to have the answer or solution to a problem. This works in marriages, as well.

I have learned since to be a better student, and to be ready to say to my fellow students, "I do not know."-Osler

55
Oh He Passes Out All the Time

Men make bad patients. Now, the wives of men will tell you the same thing. Oh yes, they will be the first to tell you that their man doesn't do well with pain. You know, a woman knows pain since they have had children, and men shouldn't complain about a prostate exam because women have been having pelvic exams since they were twenty. How about a woman's insensitivity to their male companion for having hot flashes because of his treatment for prostate cancer? "Now you'll know how I felt when I went through menopause," is the response to the patient from the wife who says it with a laugh, reinforcing the concept of men as wuses. Because of child birth, the man gets no sympathy when it comes to pain. All this, I might add, is probably appropriate; they make horrible patients in general and, in particular, awful vasectomy patients.

If a patient has a tendency to pass out with the sight of blood, seeing a needle, or the thought of a procedure on his privates, don't you think that would be something to tell the urologist *before* a vasectomy? Oh no, we have to figure it out in real time.

When the male passes out during a vasectomy here is the sequence. At the beginning of procedure he starts breathing in a loud and rhythmic fashion, he makes sure that any discomfort he is having is dully noted by the wife, who is in the room, and then you note his face is flushed.

"Do you feel warm?" is my question and is the tale tell sign of pending passing out. Then he is gone. His eyes are rolled back. He is clammy and shaking all over. The wife, unmoved by what is always dicey for me, says nonchalantly, "He does this all the time."

The patient wakes up in a few minutes and says, "Why didn't you finish the procedure while I was out?"

Rule: With men and vasectomies, if there is any history of queasiness then there is a good chance of "vasectomy vapors."

56
If I Am Going to Be Impotent Then I Am Going to Look Impotent

Okay, there is a classic urology joke that every urologist should have in his armamentarium and never fails to get a good laugh.

A man walks into a vasectomy clinic for his vasectomy all dressed up to the hilt. He has on a tuxedo, top hat and has a walking stick laden with diamonds. He was quite the dandy. He begins the sign in process with the check-in nurse. She notices his unusual attire.

"Sir, why are you so dressed up for a vasectomy," she says.

He replies, "If I am going to be impotent I want to look impotent."

Rule: Impotency relates to the inability of having an erection. Libido relates to sex drive and is dependent on testosterone which is produced by the testicles and released into the bloodstream. Fertility is having the presence of sperm in the ejaculate. A vasectomy causes sterility and does not affect testosterone. To neuter one would be cutting off the testicles which do affect testosterone. Once a male goes through puberty and the voice deepens, doing an orchiectomy (or vasectomy for that matter) will not make his voice high, i.e. talk like a girl. Most of the ejaculate is produced by the prostate and not the testicles. An orgasm is caused by the violent contraction of the external sphincter. You could explain all this to the patient so that he can defend himself from his coworkers when they find out he is having a vasectomy...or you could just tell him the joke and move on. Despite all of this and that the punch line has no medical basis and works only because of the male's lack of understanding of their genitourinary system, the joke is still universally funny and should be employed on a regular basis.

"Eunuchs do not take the gout, nor become bald."-Hippocrates

57

John There is a Stone Patient I Want You to See

I have mentioned P.K. Dixon elsewhere in this book, but he is once again a principal player in a teachable moment in my career.

I was in the office and in comes a patient in acute pain and grasping at his mid abdomen and flailing all over the place. I had been in practice about a year or so and I had no clue as to what was going on with him. I don't remember how he ended up in my office with that condition or why he didn't go to the emergency room.

I couldn't examine the abdomen because he was holding it so tight with both arms and in constant motion. We managed to put a catheter in thinking that maybe he was in retention, but the residual was small. The urine was grossly clear and positive on the dipstick for blood, but we had just catheterized him.

I thought maybe this was a dissecting aneurysm. I had never seen this before but I had heard that they were painful and mid abdominal in location. I then worry that I am missing something really serious so I call an ambulance to take him to the ER. I call Dr. Dixon and tell him the story, my concerns about a dissecting aneurysm and he agrees to see the patient when he arrives at the hospital.

Later that afternoon there is a phone call for me. It is Dr. Dixon. In a dead pan voice and in a non-condescending manor he says, "John, I have a patient in room 132 I want you to see. He is the guy you sent to the ER for me to see. He has a ureteral stone."

Embarrassing, huh? As I thought about, it dawned on me that I never see ureteral stones in the acute phase. These patients go to the ER and are treated with analgesics, and then we are called. By the time we see them they are usually comfortable and we have the CT to review and the stone has already been confirmed.

Rule: Be sure the patient doesn't have a condition you treat before you go to sending them off to another physician.

58
Two Urology Jokes

How does a man's pants fit if he has five penises?

Like a glove!

A Jewish man is walking along the beach when by chance he steps on a magic lantern. He picks it up, dusts it off and rubs it. A genie appears and states that the old man has been granted one wish, any wish that he might desire. The old man reaches deep within his chest pocket and brings out an old and wrinkled map of the Middle East.

Pointing to the Holy Land he says, "For my entire life, the land of my ancestors has been in strife and unrest. It is my wish that peace will come to my people and their neighbors and that all will live in happiness."

The genie ponders the map and says, "My dear man, as much as I would like to grant your wish, it is much too complex and longstanding an issue for me to solve for you. I am sorry. Do you have another wish?"

Dejected the old man then asks, "Can you fix it to where whenever I want to have sex with my wife she will happily comply?"

The genie again contemplates for a few minutes and then says, "May I take another look at that map?"

Genitourinary Surgeon's Motto: The difficult we handle right away; the impossible takes a little longer.

"Life is short and the Art is long; the occasion fleeting; experience fallacious; judgment difficult."-Osler

59
The Heartbreak of Lithiasis

As a urologist, you get to know some patients better than others. The prostate cancer patient who has been treated and you follow up with a couple times a year becomes familiar to you. The BPH patient, on maximum meds, whom you see to refill medicines and check his prostate, also becomes a "friend patient." The most familiar and often the most difficult, however, is the recurrent stone patient. When I am seeing a patient in follow up after a ureteroscopic stone extraction, the last thing I do is look at the CT for residual renal stones and say to the patient, "Let's see what the future holds for you."

These poor patients; they go through the horrible pain and inconvenience of the stones, the radiation used in making the diagnosis, the treatment and then are at risk at any time for the other foot to drop. Over the years I have asked patients what to them was the most painful thing they had ever endured. I have had three knee injuries and subsequent surgeries and I thought that was pretty bad. I had a patient one time who had had a baby, knee surgery, been shot, and had passed a stone. By far this patient stated that the stone pain was the worst.

One day I am in my office and a frequent flyer stone patient is seeing me in follow up and told me he wanted to show me something.

"Doc, I want you to see something to show you how much I appreciate all you have done for me over the years." At this point he takes his shirt off to reveal a chest with about a hundred tattoos all over it. Just below the left nipple and above a yellow Tweety Bird was a stethoscope surrounded by about ten small stones and this inscription:

"Dr. McHugh-Stone Man."

"You shouldn't have done that," I say. "That is permanent; you liking me in a few years may not be."

Just a few weeks before, he had been in the ER and my partner was unsure if he was a seeker (That's another thing. Recurrent stone patients have to continually ask for pain medicine, and are sometimes suspected as seekers) and did not give him the amount or the type of narcotic he wanted.

"If I see your partner again, I am going to whip his ass," he says to me. All I can think about now is seeing my name tattooed on his chest and his being disappointed with my care one day, all the while being stuck with me below his nipple and beside Tweety Bird.

Over the years, this particular patient came to loath stents. Here's something I have learned: *stents are blessing and a curse to the patient.* If a patient has had pain from a non-infected but obstructive stone and you only put a stent in and nothing else, they will tolerate the stent well. If they weren't having much pain or you use a stent post-ureteroscopy, it has the potential of being a miserable experience for the patient. The patient who has had a bad experience with a stent will not forget it. This patient was that class of patient and as well had no hesitation in saying so.

"Doc, I'll let you get this stone, but I don't want no stent. *Do not* put a stent in me."

"I cannot promise that. If I can't get the stone or if getting it is difficult, it will be best for you to have one, temporarily."

"I don't want a stent."

"Well, then I can't do your surgery."

"Promise me you'll do a stent as an absolute last resort."

"I promise," I said considering this a huge concession.

Years later I performed a percutaneous nephrostolithotomy on this patient for an upper pole stone, and the initial placement of the wire by the radiologist transgressed the pleural cavity and irrigation fluids entered his chest requiring a chest tube.

"If I ever meet that radiologist I'm going to whip his ass," he told me post operatively.

Rule: Once the patient tries to exert ownership and dictate the patient- physician relationship, the urologist must nip it in the bud early on or find the patient another doctor. It just doesn't work that way and no good can come of it.

"I tawt I taw a pudney tone!"

60
The Prostate Exam-An Art Form?

The rectal exam: the patient doesn't want it done, and the doctor can be easily persuaded not to do it.

Oh you know the jokes, "Doc, was that your left hand on my shoulder or you right hand while you did my exam. Wait a minute! You had both hands!" I have had patients tell me this joke a thousand times. I smile like I've never heard it.

How about this one: The urologist examines the patient's prostate and tells him he suspects cancer and recommends a biopsy. The patient says, "Hold on doc, not so fast, I want a second opinion."

The urologist then says, "Bend over again and I'll check you with two fingers."

We had an attending that told us to take care when performing a rectal exam, "Boys, the urologist elevates the rectal exam to an art form."

There may be some truth to that. We do use a lot of KY and that helps. We put mild pressure on the inferior rim of the anal verge and that does tend relax the sphincter. We know what we are feeling for and so the exam should take less time. Maybe there is some truth that urologists take an uncomfortable situation for the male and an uncomfortable exam for the male and make it better than if performed by a rank amateur. Why shouldn't we take the time and effort to make our exam better?

Rule: If the patient doesn't complain that you used too much KY, or that it seems to be reproducing itself as he cleans himself off, then you didn't use enough. You need to use the "urological" amount of KY jelly.

The prostate is the Rodney Dangerfield of medicine; it don't get no respect.

"One finger in the throat and one in the rectum makes a good diagnostician."-Osler

61
Good News, Bad News, and Washing Machines

A patient comes into the doctor's office for the results of some tests and biopsies. The doctor enters the exam room and sits with the patient.

"I have some good news and some bad news for you sir. Which would you like me to tell you first?"

The patient after some consideration says, "Give me the good news first."

"Well Mr. Smith, you have one week to live."

The patient is devastated initially but then is confused.

"If that is the good news, then what on earth is the bad news?"

"I am so sorry," says the doctor.

"I meant to tell you last week."

Rule: It is not what you say but how you say it. Timing is everything.

There was this couple who used the word "playing washing machine" as a euphemism for having sex. One night the husband cuddles up to the wife and says, "Do you want to play washing machine?"

The wife says, "I am sorry honey, but I have a headache."

The couple then rolls their separate ways to go to sleep. After about fifteen minutes, the wife feeling guilty says, "Honey, if you want to play washing machine we can. I feel much better now."

The husband responds, "That's okay. It was a small load and I did it by hand!"

Rule: It is never a bad idea to have a plan B or an alternate approach.

62
Your Magazines Are All Out of Date

We recently converted to a new EMR system and one nice feature is that it tells you how long it's been since the patient arrived in the office. I guess it helps me a bit; I mean how much I grovel about apologizing to the patient about being late or keeping him waiting.

So the following is an interchange with a patient with a list of grievances. As he begins, I note that he checked in 23 minutes before me entering the room.

"I am sorry to have kept you waiting. How are you today?"

"What station is that you are playing on your intercom system? Not only is it not appropriate for a doctor's office, it has static all through the song. You need to change that."

As I begin to ask a question, he interrupts, "Your telephone system lies. It says that you should listen to all the options before making a selection because it has recently changed. I know for a fact that it has not changed. Don't you think you should have magazines that are for men and ones that are not so out of date?"

At this point I sit down and pretend to be taking notes; I feign interest.

"Another thing is that a member of your staff referred to me as "honey" and I found that unprofessional and condescending. She was chewing gum for heaven's sake!"

"Well, Mr. Smith, I am truly sorry about that. I will speak to my office manager regarding those issues. I do have, however, the results of your prostate biopsy. It shows that you have a moderately aggressive prostate cancer."

At that moment, the less than the desirable nuances of my office became glaringly less important to him.

Rule: When patients seemingly are acting in an inappropriate manor, it might be a manifestation of anxiety regarding their health. And for this reason, and as hard as it may be for the doctor, they get a pass. As Osler said of nurses, "To her virtues we have been exceedingly kind-tongues have dropped manna in their description. To her faults-well let us be blind."

63
Blood Clots and Gummy Bears

Attempts at humor can work for you or against you. Humor in medicine is tricky, and I have messed it up more than once trying to be funny. Oh sure, I did it in the guise of making the patient and family laugh but humor makes me feel better also; it helps me get through the day. Elsewhere the quote about, "It's not what you say but how you say it...and timing is everything" is used for other subjects but there is no better application, or lack of, than what follows.

There was a patient that I inherited (The proverbial shit baton) who had gross hematuria. He was in the hospital on overhead irrigation. He had the TURP two weeks previously and two subsequent procedures to stop the bleeding by two other urologists. No sooner did the 7 A.M. on call start time begin when I am barraged with phone calls about "something has got to be done!" Case management was involved.

I take the guy to the operating room and luckily find the bleeding point anteriorly in the prostatic fossa underneath a fold of unresected prostate tissue. Even a blind hog will find an acorn from time to time. The urine was immediately off the drip and is clear as a bell; I was proud of myself. I cured somebody of something.

I begin to tell the family how well the patient is doing, but the only thing the family members want to tell me is the rehash of the two week history of how the patient was passing clots. Each passed clot was described very intricately; the color, the size, a picture of one on a phone and then to top that off, they even have saved one in a handkerchief. There was a picture of a clot in a toilet. I wanted to talk about how I had stopped the bleeding when two other urologists had failed and be in the present. Then I stepped in it.

"You know the patient and family put a lot of emphasis on clots from the bladder, however, if they are not associated with not being able to void, they don't cause much harm. When patients hear the term clot or see bladder clots they tend to think of the clots that go to the heart or form in the legs. These are different."

As I was speaking I failed to read the faces of the six or so family members assembled to be with a loved one who had been dealing with gross hematuria for two weeks and their fourth time in the operating room waiting area waiting to speak to the surgeon.

"Clots and family members being concerned about clots, happen so often I have a little skit I do about them. Everybody wants to describe the clot but a description is not medically necessary or relevant. So I'll pretend I want to know every detail. I ask about what shade of purple was the clot, does it look more like a plastic worm you would fish with or a gummy bear? You see, a clot in the bladder is a glob of blood, but when it is extruded through the urethra, it changes form from a gummy bear to a gummy worm. I also ask about how did it feel when it came out, what did it look like in the toilet, did it make a sound, and did it float or sink? You know clots in the bladder behave much like a bouillon cube; you can have bloody urine but no active bleeding because the clot is just dissolving and coloring the urine."

It was the triple whammy of bad. It was *what* I said, it was *how* I said it, and my *timing* was horrible. My monologue resulted in complete silence and elicited disgust, both old and young, by all in the room. Not only had I been insensitive about a loved one who had suffered so, they perceived that I had made fun of them as well.

From this point on, despite my apologies and attempts at an explanation, the wife could not bring herself to look or speak to me. My partner had done the original surgery so in follow up they saw him. I was at check out when they were there to see him and this time neither the patient nor the wife could muster even making eye contact with me.

You would think that after 25 years of practicing urology that I would have been able to read my audience better.

Rule: On the other hand, they could have laughed and appreciated my humor. Maybe it was my delivery. Next time I'll...
"Use humor with patients and families judiciously-you must stop all attempts at humor after the first blank look."-Leo Gordon.

64
"Cold Snap"

Everybody knows about the prostate, particularly prostatitis, being sensitive to certain foods that are spicy or acidic, but what about the weather?

One fall in the urology clinic, we began to notice an increase in the men presenting in urinary retention; they were showing up in droves.

One of the residents, during rounds one day, mentioned this observation to Dr. Witherington, the Chairman of Urology, and his response I have never forgotten.

"Boys, the prostate is very sensitive to a change in the weather. When prostatism evolves into retention in the colder months, there has probably been a cold snap."

Rule: This does not mean, however, that the prostate can predict the weather, or that your finger in examining it is a weather vane. (Did you know another name for a weather vane is a weathercock?) In other words, if the prostate aches, it doesn't necessarily mean that it is going to rain. Your joints and the prostate are different that way.

"All diseases occur at all seasons of the year, but certain of them are more apt to occur and be exacerbated at certain seasons."-Hippocrates.

"Whoever is desirous of prosecuting his medical studies on a right plan must pay a good deal of attention to the different seasons of the year and their respective influence."-Hippocrates

65
May I Bless You Doctor McHugh?

A word to the wise: if you suspect urine under pressure (in the old days we called it a "hydronephrotic drip" if urine came out of a ureteral catheter in a steady stream), with or without known infection, you best get the hell in and get the hell out.

A very pleasant woman presented to my office, after having been seen in the E.R., with a several day history right flank pain and not feeling well. No temperature, minimal white count and a seven mm mid-ureteral stone. The urine was clear. She and the husband wanted something done.

The next day, with preoperative antibiotics on board, I planned to remove the stone if it were easy and if not place a stent. Well, a glide wire would not go past the stone so I used a flexible ureteroscope to visualize the stone and manipulate the wire by it, replaced the flexible scope with a rigid scope, removed the stone and placed a stent. This took about forty-five minutes.

In the recovery room she became septic. All of her parameters went to hell in a hand basket and she was placed in intensive care. I consulted everyone I could think of and she was placed on two types of broad spectrum antibiotics, pressers, and all of other things that sick people get. Two days later the blood cultures reveal an E.coli strain that is not sensitive to the antibiotics she was on; the one with the best sensitivity was one I had never heard of or used before. She slowly gets better, but the new antibiotic caused an issue with her heart rhythm, gave her extensive mouth and lip blisters, and to top it all off, clumps of hair begin to fall out. With time she got better, moved to the floor, and then discharged.

A few week later in the office she was in good spirits, had cut her hair real short to deemphasize the hair loss and all the blisters were now crusting over.

"Doctor McHugh, did you know that I died the night you put me into intensive care? I saw a bright light and above me were members of my church holding hands in the shape of a rainbow, and I was floating up to them. Someone said that God was not ready for me yet and I floated back down and then woke up."

I listened, mesmerized. I have heard of this type of thing but never had spoken to someone personally who had experienced it. The thing is that in my mind I had caused the issue in the first place. Yes, that's right. I felt responsible for what she had been through; if I had just put the stent in and come back another day, or chosen different antibiotics, she'd probably done fine.

"Also Dr. McHugh, I wanted to tell you also that I am moving to Minnesota; my husband is from there, and he wants to be near his family. So, thank you for all you did for me."
She then stands and hugs me and continues to hold my hand.

"Dr. McHugh, may I bless you?"

It was here that I lost it. I am easy to cry anyway, but this was over the top. We are now holding hands and crying together.

"Of course you can, I mean, please. I need all the blessings I can get!"

Rule: A urologist should always have an a heightened sense of awareness. A completely obstructing stone with infection can be associated with no significant hydronephrosis, clean urine, no fever or elevated white count and yet will rear up and bite your ass if you ain't thinking.

Patient: "Dr. McHugh, how are you today?"
McHugh: "Not the best...but I'm blessed."

"The practice of medicine is an art, not a trade; a calling, not a business; a calling in which your heart will be exercised equally with your head."-Osler

"The greatest of mistake in the treatment of diseases is that there are physicians for the body and physicians for the soul, although the two cannot be separated."-Plato

Just as a parent is only as happy as his unhappiest child, so too should the physician be only as happy as his sickest patient, particularly if his surgery perpetrated the issue.

66

The Dick Pool

Until the fifth grade, my family lived in Columbus, Georgia. We lived on a dirt road adjacent to a nice neighborhood, which in turn, was near the Moose Club. I could cut through that neighborhood, go through a patch of woods and end up at the Moose Club in about 20 minutes.

I remember walking barefoot in the summer to swimming practice, and how my feet would be tender at the beginning of the summer and would be tough as nails by the end of summer. I never wore shoes. All of my four brothers were on the Moose Club Swim team and we all were pretty good at it. There was only one other guy my age that I couldn't beat. Other than him, I won the vast majority of my events. A lifelong dream of mine was to have a house with a swimming pool that had a lap lane.

Zoom forward to me living in Gainesville and building a home in which will have a pool with a lap lane. The shape of the pool and incorporating a lap lane was more of a task than I had imagined. We got a company out of Atlanta to design and build the pool. The problem with the design was how to incorporate something for our three children, yet accommodate me as well. I distinctly remember being given a large sheet of paper with at least twenty shapes of pools, each with a lap lane. The one I elected to use was based on the recommendations of the guy that did our landscaping. He liked the design best that looked like a gun, an oval shape at one end with the lap lane extending from it. The shape conformed to the backyard and porch and also allowed for a twenty-five foot long lane. We even planned to have tile embedded in the lap lane to make it look official. The depth of the lane allowed for flip turns.

So, I am over at the house as it is being built and the gunite is being poured for the pool, and I am just looking around and taking it in. It was exciting; a new home and a pool with my very own lap lane.

That is, until it dawns on me that the pool looks like a penis. What I had gone to such pains to have and design looks like a urologist had purposely designed a dick pool. I have yet to hear the end of it. Having two dachshunds (wiener dogs) did not help matters.

Rule: Sometimes seeing the diagnosis requires appraising the situation from different angles and perspectives. Or as you'll note in what follows, seeing with a little imagination, and an oblique view, at a distance...

"Half of us are blind, few of us feel and we are all deaf."-Osler

Years ago my hiking group and I canoed a stretch of the Missouri River that Lewis and Clark had traversed with the Corps of Discovery. This section highlights the Upper Missouri River Breaks National Monument. In "The Journals of Lewis and Clark" Lewis describes the hills and river cliffs of this area as "exhibiting a most romantic appearance." I mention this because I have always loved Lewis' description of the cliffs and how what he wrote could apply to physicians viewing the various diseases we encounter daily. It also applies to how we view our patients, our colleagues, our family and life. Enjoy.

"The water, in the course of time, descending from those hills and plains, on either side of the river, has trickled down the soft sand cliffs and worn it into a thousand grotesque figures, which, **with the help of a little imagination, and an oblique view, at a distance** *are made to represent elegant ranges of lofty freestone buildings, having their parapets well stocked in statuary."-May 1805- Meriwether Lewis*

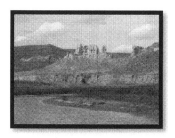

67
Polychronotopic, Farmers and Hat Pins

Patients with recurrent low-grade transitional cell carcinoma of the bladder can be a tricky bunch to treat. If these patients have been on intravesical therapy, just keeping up with the treatments they have had and determining future treatments is difficult. The follow-up of cystoscopy every three months for two years, then cystoscopy every six months for two years, and then yearly if no recurrence, is a lot to bear if you are the patient. And then, you throw in a recurrence and you have to start the whole process all over, all the while worrying that there is some deeper element of the disease in the muscle that you just haven't sampled yet. It's tricky.

Patients who have gotten to the six month follow-up and then have a recurrence most likely will be told he needs to start over and consider a second course of BCG or a maintenance type plan potentially with a different agent. Add to the mix that this patient has a 20 some odd year history of smoking.

"Why can't you cure me of this doc?"

"I know this is frustrating Mr. Smith. You see the smoking made certain toxins touch your bladder all over for many years and so when we treat one cancer another pops up in a different area."

"But I quit smoking five years ago."

"Well it takes about 15 years for bladder cancer to show up in someone who has smoked. These cancers are the result of a cigarette a long time ago."

"Well you have looked in my bladder about 10 times, put all that medicine in there and I am still getting the cancer. Why can't you just take it out?"

You get the picture. If you have a mole on your arm and the doctor removes it, it is gone and you can look at the area every day to be sure it doesn't return. The concept of polychronotopic is not an easy one.

"You know how you have seen people who have been treated for skin cancer on their face. They will have one treated and another one will pop up on the other side of the face. Like farmers who have been exposed to the sun for a long time, so too your bladder has been exposed to the toxins in cigarettes for a long time. You bladder is like the farmer's face."

Rule: No sir, the cancer did not come back. A new one occurred in a different location. The one we treated is gone. I understand completely if you would like a second opinion about this as I know it has been frustrating for you.

I had a patient who had low grade papillary TCC in at least 85% of his bladder. He was on Coumadin for a heart condition which complicated his urologic care. It took several resections, each with the process of weaning off and then weaning back on the Coumadin, to render him free of disease. His wife is about five feet tall and quite the spitball. She was related to Pope Innocent X (1574-1655) and her grandfather was a urologist in New York in the early 1900s. She had given me a paper he'd written about removing a 9 inch pin from the urethra of man's penis that had been in a journal at that time. I got to know the patient and the wife very well throughout the course of his treatments.

"Doctor McHugh, I want to show you something."
In an intricate and old fashioned case, she shows me a small hat pin topped with a pearl and adorned with other jewels. It was very pretty.

"This is a segment of the pin my grandfather removed from that man's urethra in 1909. My grandmother had the pin shortened at Tiffany and gifted it with the pearl on top to my grandfather. Pretty huh?"

If that pin could talk.

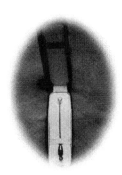

A man and his wife were at an office visit with the urologist.

The wife says, "Something must be done. My husband's penis drags the floor and he is always stepping on it."

The urologist examines the man and sure enough the length of the penis has not been overstated and it is black and blue from being trampled upon.

The wife said, "Doc, can you correct this?"

The urologist says, "Yes I can."

After the surgery the urologist goes out to the waiting room to speak to the man's wife.

"Everything went fine. I was able to remove enough of the penis safely to have it be about at the level of his knees. This should correct the problem."

Aghast, the woman replies, "I did not want you to shorten his penis. I wanted you to make his legs longer! "

Rule: When it comes to circumcisions be sure to measure twice and cut once.

68
The Last Guy I Told Joined the Other Urology Group in Town

There are some things we do in urology, the concept of which, is difficult for both the doctor and the patient to grasp. For example, "Where does sperm go after a vasectomy?" or "If the stone is near my bladder, why am I hurting in my back?" These are good, but my favorite is this one.

After explaining the procedure and expected course of having the Greenlight Laser done, it is not uncommon for the patient to stand, go to the anatomic chart on the door and point to the prostate.

"Two questions for you doc: the urethra here goes through the prostate, right? How are you going to make the hole bigger in the prostate without destroying the urethra? Then, also, how will you get prostate tissue out of the bladder when you are done?"

Well I could say, "Mr. Smith, I could tell you but I'd have to kill you." But I don't anymore. I have a better response.

"Mr. Smith, that is a good question. I would tell you how I do that, but it is somewhat of a trade secret. One time I told a patient how I do it and the next thing I know he's working for the other urology group in town."

Rule: Just as magicians should never tell the method of their tricks, so too are there some urology tricks you should keep close to the vest. Now the example above is not one of them, but the complexity of performing an ESWL is, and should never be disclosed.

Urologist: "Do you see it? 1 cm and UPJ."
Lithotripsy technician: "Yes. Do you want the rate fast or slow?"
Urologist: "Fast."
Thirty five minutes later-Urologist: "Did it change?"
Lithotripsy technician: "Yes."
Urologist "22 and 3000?"
Lithotripsy technician: "24 and 3000."
Urologist: "Thank you."

69
Gilding the Lily

Dr. Witherington used this phrase often in a variety of circumstances. It is a corollary of "the enemy of good is better" or "why do more if it is not necessary" sayings. It is like a customer agreeing to buy an item for five dollars. The deal is done, there is no more need for the salesman to negotiate or lower the price; he needs to be quite and stop.

If you are doing a plication for Peyronies disease and the penis is straight with two sutures on each side, why place more? You've fragmented and removed 95% of a mid-ureteral stone, do you spend another fifteen minutes trying to get 100% of the stone? In doing ESWL the stone is non-visible at 1000 shocks; do you do an additional 1000 for good measure? Finally, in doing a TURP, you have created a very nice channel that is clearly patent, yet you feel you need to do just a little more. Uh oh, that last cut resulted in bleeding and requires further fulguration and irrigation of tissue and prolongs the procedure by fifteen minutes. And for what?

Gilding the lily is doing something that is not necessary and over the course of the day economy of motion by the urologist will save time and keep you out of unnecessary trouble.

Rule: "To gild refined gold, to paint the lily, to throw a perfume on the violet, to smooth the ice, or add another hue unto the rainbow, or with taper-light to seek the beauteous eye of heaven to garnish, is wasteful and ridiculous excess." Shakespeare *King John* 1595

"In life's perspective we seniors are apt to resent that the rising generation should work out its own salvation in ways that are not always our ways, and with thoughts that are not always our thoughts. One thing is in our power, to admix in due proportions with their present somewhat rickety bill of fare the more solid nourishment of the English Bible and of Shakespeare."-Osler

The enemy of good is better.

The art of knowing when to stop.

70
Coup de Grace

I hesitate adding this chapter for fear someone will judge me, but I have decided to press forward. Another favorite phrase of our chief Dr. Witherington was *coup de grace*, or the last blow. You can use it for anything: that last parameter that falters and assures the demise of a patient, that final tap of the laser that renders the stone to dust, or that last vestige of tissue that keeps an organ in the body before its extirpation.

Although most radical prostatectomies are now done robotically, before 2007, the most common method was the open Walsh prostatectomy. This procedure revolutionized the removal of the prostate and this, in conjunction of the PSA, resulted in urologists doing a bunch of prostatectomies. For years, it was the number one open procedure I did, and, consequently, I became very good at performing it. Ain't saying I was the best, but twern't many better.

As you know, it is not unusual to have a new scrub tech or student assisting in surgery. If I had a new member who had never done a prostatectomy with me, as a rite of passage, I did my coup de grace move on them. Toward the end of the procedure and after the urethra and bladder had been dissected free, all that remained were the limbs of the seminal vesicles. The foley would still be going through the prostate and elevated upward to facilitate the final dissection. When I would get to point where all that remained was the last leg of the seminal vesicles and it was cross clamped, this is where the "trick" began.

I give the foley, which is now reflected on itself and under elastic tension, to the student and say, "tension please...just a little more please." As the foley is pulled much like a rubber band, I cut the last strand of tissue holding the seminal vesicles. This results in the prostate springing up out of the wound with the foley and the shocked student thinking he has pulled it out. The entire team, who have been in on it before, acts surprised and concerned that something bad has happened, much to the chagrin of the student.

"I said tension! Goodness graciousness, I did not say to yank it out!"

Rule: Everything has its coup de grace. You just have to recognize it.

"Hilarity and good humor, a breezy cheerfulness, a nature "sloping toward the southern side," as Lowell has it [referring to the sunny side, from "An Epistle to George William Curtis" by James Russell Lowell (1819-1891)], help enormously both in the study and in the practice of medicine. To many of a somber and sour disposition it is hard to maintain good spirits amid the trial and tribulations of the day, and yet it is an unpardonable mistake to go about among patients with a long face."-Osler

Every one of the "Big Four," as they are known at Hopkins, was a character, a larger-than-life personality: pathologist William Henry Welch, a stout bachelor whose favorite pastime was a week of swimming, carnival rides and five-dessert dinners in Atlantic City; surgeon William Stewart Halsted, whose severity with students masked an almost debilitating shyness; **internist William Osler, king of pranks;** *and gynecologist Howard Kelly, snake collector and evangelical saver of souls.-Hopkinsmedicine.org*

71

It Takes a Smart Doctor to Know When Someone Is Dying

When I was a surgical intern in Augusta, Georgia, in 1982, I was making rounds with a vascular surgery service. My group, which included interns, residents, nurses, and the attending physician, were standing around an unfortunate patient in the intensive care unit. This patient had tubes everywhere, was on many medicines, recently had had one leg removed from complications of diabetes, and now had developed some redness on a small area of his left arm. The chief resident began to spout off numerous options regarding what could be done, listed several diagnostic studies and lab tests that could be ordered, additional medications to institute, and then delineated the surgical options.

All standing there including me were impressed by the litany of therapeutic options the chief resident delivered. After a pause, the attending physician said, "Harvey, have you ever seen the firefighters on TV fighting those fires in California?" The chief resident, somewhat puzzled, said, "Yes sir, I have." The attending continued in a prolonged Southern drawl, "You see them there with all that garb on and a backpack with a little hose shooting out a tiny stream of water at the base of one of those big California trees that is smoking, and all the while you see the forest fire behind them just raging out of control." The chief resident, who is just one step and weeks away from being a "real" doctor, and all the others assembled there just stood in silence trying to make sense of these obtuse words of wisdom and how they may be related to the patient we were all observing. After what seemed to be a long pause, with the attending physician peering at the patient and all of us peering at him, he said, "Harvey, let's just leave Mr. Johnson alone, why don't we?" From *The Decision*

Rule: The trick is knowing who to let die and who you try to keep alive...and timing is everything.
"Dying is not difficult, yielding is impossible."-Sydenham

72
A Silk Purse out of Sow's Ear

When it comes to advising a patient to have an inflatable penile prosthesis placed, you'd better make sure it is the last resort. I don't care how hard they push you to skip to that treatment option. You should use the neurosurgeon's technique of making it very clear that "We are operating on your back because conservative measures have not worked, and I can make no guarantees regarding outcome" or "This procedure destroys the natural ability of the penis to get erect; you can't go back once we do this."

But this is only the start. You see, some patients think that the prosthesis makes things bigger. You can say it ten times, but they don't hear it and they don't hear that the head does not engorge and the girth will be less. Initially, you should try to talk them out of it, because there is no wrath like the impotent man scorned. If they persist, know the downside risk and that you are only promising a firm penis and that is all, you may want to proceed. Make sure they know about the potential for prolonged post-operative pain after insertion. Oh, and don't forget that there may be an infection and that the prosthesis may need to be removed and, if removed, you may not be able to put another one in. And since the cavernosa are now sclerotic, happy days will not be here again.

After all this and every *i* is dotted and all *t*'s are crossed, you successfully put in the prosthesis, and you are now showing the patient how to cycle it up a month later. It turns out the patient has poor hand to eye coordination, and this is a task that he can't master in one office visit. But even now, this isn't the kicker.

"Doc, my penis was much bigger than this before you put this in. I bet it is at least an inch and half shorter," he says as his wife, who is in the room as well, nods in agreement.

Rule: You can make a penis firm; you can't make a purse from a sow's ear.
Father to son: I said I'd take you fishing...I didn't say we'd catch fish.

73
What You Say Ain't Always What They Hear

There are certain phrases and things that patients say and do that you'll hear over and over again during the course of your practice. For instance, our exam tables have a small foot platform at the end which is designed to help patients get up to and sit on the exam table. Invariably, at the time of a rectal exam, as the patient begins to unbutton his pants, he'll see the platform and will try to kick it in before bending over. The platform is not in the patient's way, but for some reason, this is a response I have seen a thousand times and results in me saying, "That's okay, it can stay out."

You'll hear from patients often saying that cancer of the prostate is "the slow growing kind" and you'll see the patient rub his lumbosacral area and say, "My kidneys hurt right here." The next one is a common one too, but with a twist that even impressed me when I witnessed it. Patients with kidney stones will ask, "A buddy told me to drink beer and that will flush the stone out." I'll say that beer won't hurt but it is more about increased hydration than the type of liquid consumed.

I am seeing a patient I treated for kidney stones years ago. He tells me that since I saw him last, he had remarried. "I met her at the church where I am the choir director; my wife is in the choir and that is how we met. I want to introduce her to you."

"Honey, this is Dr. McHugh. He is the one that recommended that I have two beers before breakfast each morning to prevent kidney stones," he says as the new wife looks at me with questioning eyes. I don't blame her; I have never told anyone that.

I just smile and nod my head and think, "This guy is good." "Well, staying well hydrated is important with stones," I muster.

Rule: People tend to do what works. Who am I to argue? By the looks of it, this patient has not had a stone for over four years.

74
Kill Them with Kindness

As it pertains to having messed up or as one might say, having achieved a less than desirable result, you must sometimes kill 'em with kindness.

"Dr. McHugh do you still need to see me so often?"

"Well Mr. Smith what do you think? Do you feel you have improved enough to maybe lengthen the follow-up time frame?"

I had this patient one time that had both a long urethra and a long prostatic urethra. You may not believe this but the regular instruments barely reached the bladder neck. In addition, he had a large median lobe of the prostate which exacerbated the issue of the intended TURP. The first time I attempted the procedure, my performance was somewhat less than desired; replete with an incomplete resection and prolonged post-operative bleeding and the need for prolonged irrigation. He eventually was well enough to go home, but I told him of the inadequate length of the instruments and that he most probably would need another procedure with longer instruments if what I had just done did not improve his stream adequately. Well you guessed it, the stream did not improve and he continued to have hematuria, forcing my hand at another TURP. I call the Storz representative and see if there exists a "long set" of TURP instruments and find out that there did exist such a set. I ask him to let me borrow them and then reschedule the procedure. With the new instruments the procedure is still a struggle but proceeded much better. A nice channel was fashioned and bleeding was controlled adequately. The procedure was done on the Friday before Mother's day and my partner was on call for the weekend. I see the patient Friday evening and tell him that I will be out of town visiting my mother. I tell him the on call doctor will take care of him over the weekend and, if appropriate, send him home.

I go to see my mother and return the following Monday. On Tuesday I get a call from a nurse on the urology floor.

"Dr. McHugh, will you be seeing Mr. Smith today? He wants to go home."

"Is he still in the hospital?"

"Yes, no one has seen him since Friday. He wife is angry and wants to know when a doctor will be seeing him."

For whatever reason my partner did not see the patient over the weekend and I assumed he had gone home. So this patient, who was post-surgical, was not seen by a physician for three days in the hospital. Basically, a lawsuit waiting to happen if any else untoward comes of the procedure I had performed. I rush over to the hospital and apologize profusely and arrange for his discharge and follow up in the office. Sometimes we just need a little help from the patient. Why couldn't he have said something to the nurse earlier?

"My wife says I should get another doctor. She says they have better doctors in Atlanta. She doesn't drive and getting back up here to see you is hard."

I say," Where do you live? I'll come to see you at your house."

A week later I arrive at this patient's house and follow up with him in his kitchen.

He said to me, "You didn't bring me flowers? How is your mother doing?"

I went back two weeks later to confirm again that all was well, which it was, and then he agreed to see me once a year in the office.

I saw him many times over the ensuing years and he became a favorite patient of mine and we had fun recounting the Mother's Day affair.

Rule: When a patient has a wife that wants him to see another urologist, for any reason, encourage it. They are doing you a favor.

Wife of patient: "Well, if you are not going to do the procedure that I want you to do, I am going to get my husband another doctor!"
Urologist: "May I give you some names?" (The competing urologist you like the least comes to mind.)

75
Trains, Perspective, and Mr. Tomanek

I remember Mr. Tomanek for many reasons, but for two in particular. He loved trains. He lived in the mountains just south of Helen, Georgia, and built a garage specifically for his model trains and all the stuff that goes with that. I looked at pictures of the new additions at each office visit. The other thing about him was the relationship between him and his wife. When I first met them, she had just had a base of tongue resection and all the facial and neck incisions were healing. It affected how she talked and it affected her facial expressions. I was blessed to have worked with them for over 15 years. In the beginning, he was strong and she was sickly. Then they were about the same and then he had a stroke making him weak and her strong. And man was she strong. She became, over time, the dominant part of the relationship. She did right by him.

What I have described, I have witnessed many times in my 25 year plus career; the ebb and flow of a relationship and the alternating pattern of health that accompanies it over time. Mrs. Tomanek seemed to become stronger as she aged and Mr. Tomanek deteriorated equally in reverse. Mr. Tomanek had a stent that we exchanged every six months because of a ureteral stricture secondary to repeated bladder cancer resections. In time Mr. Tomanek became home bound and on Hospice and we elected to just leave the stent be.

One day there is a phone call from Mrs. Tomanek, "Dr. McHugh, Frank is having a lot of blood in his urine and I was hoping you could just remove the stent and leave it out."
"Sure," I say, "when do you want to come to have it done?"
"Can you come here and remove it; at our house?"

I paused. There was no question that I wouldn't accommodate Mr. Tomanek, I was just going through my head the logistics of having all the stuff I'd need to take the stent out and if I could do it by myself with her help.

"When do you want me to be there?"

My nurse and I packed up the irrigation fluid, the graspers, the light source, betadine and the flexible light source and I was on my way. I knew the area in and about Helen but the key was to turn just before Helen at a roadside vegetable market. As I turned on to the road, I said to myself that I would be stopping there on the way back to get some tomatoes.

When I arrived, Mrs. Tomanek, who had to be almost eighty, was at the top of a twenty-foot ladder adjusting a wire that was attached to her satellite system. It was crazy seeing this; I had my camera and took a picture of her up there.

She takes me inside and, in an old-fashioned bedroom replete with generations of pictures, was Mr. Tomanek in his bed gazing listlessly out the window.

I set up my stuff and luckily remove the stent without an issue. I give them the stent as a souvenir. "Look, it's a boy." Mrs. Tomanek gives me a blue wooden train engine. "He'd want you to have this," she says.

I never saw Mr. Tomanek again. I may have seen Mrs. Tomanek once since.

Rule: One of the beauties of years of experience is perspective. You develop a feel for how things play out because you have witnessed the evolution of relationships just as you have various diseases. This in turn makes you a better doctor and adds texture to your acumen.

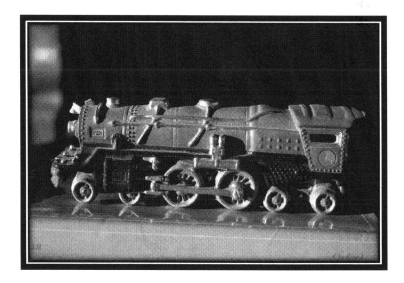

76
Will You Please Give the Phone to Your Husband?

Being on call becomes much more laborious as you mature in your urological journey. Besides the threat of having to go into the hospital at an inopportune time, there are those pesky phone calls. A "name and number" call from the hospital operator results in a series of predictable events.

You have the operator connect you to the patient, but the line is busy. You see, if you are the patient and you have called the hospital for the doctor, then that is a good time to catch up with a friend or order out. It is understandable, right? You try again, which in turn means calling the hospital. You can't call with your cell phone because then the patient will have your personal number, so you have to go through the operator and then wait for the patient to answer, that is if he is not already talking with someone else. If you are connected to the patient and they want something for pain, then you have to sort out if the request is legitimate or not. If you agree to call in a pain medicine, then you are setting yourself up for a similar call the next time you are on call.

Pain medicine requesters have a way of being repeat offenders. If you suggest that the patient go to the ER, then you'll hear about the inconvenience and expense of this and "Can't you just call something in this time?" If you don't comply with the request and the patient does go to the ER, then you get yet another call regarding this patient and that he or she has already had five CT scans this year and they have shown stones in the kidney but no obstruction. What to do?

But that is not my story; I want to describe the family member who wants to relay the information about the patient and his problem. "I am calling for my husband. He had a stone removed three days ago and is peeing blood."

"Does he have a stent?" you ask.

"Honey, did the doctor say anything about a stent?" There is a pause. You hear something being said in the distance. She repeats the question to the husband. Your phone goes off; it is the hospital ER with questions about the patient requesting pain medication you spoke to earlier.

Here's what you have to do. It is better to do it from the get go, because the question to the wife from you, the question from the wife to the patient, from the patient to the wife, and then the wife to you will go on into infinity if you don't nip it in the bud. Go to the source.

"Will you please give the phone to your husband?"

Rule: You need to hear it from the horse's mouth. Although family members want to make it about them and how they have been inconvenienced by their family member's disease and how much they love the patient and want the best for them...it is not about them. Bring them back to the source...it is about the patient and not the family member attempting to be relevant and the ostentatious show of affection.

A man is at the door to leave for a business trip. His wife, very attractive and dressed in a provocative night gown, is kissing him good-bye when the phone rings. The wife attempts to get it but the husband is closer and he picks up the phone.

"Hello? Yes. Well as a matter of fact I am travelling today and have seen the weather report. The temperature will be about 70 today and partly cloudy. The weatherman said that a cold front is coming in and that we can expect showers tomorrow, but by the weekend the conditions for the beaches will be very pleasant. Sure, you are quite welcome, glad I could help. Have a nice day."

The wife with an anxious look of concern asks, "Is everything all right honey? Who was that?"

The husband says as he was leaving, "I don't know. It was just some guy wanting to know if the coast was clear."

77

Friends and Family Get the Worst Treatment and the Worst Results

It used to be that you could see a family member, friend or colleague and just file the charges as "insurance only." This way you were able to show deference to the person while being reimbursed for your time and supplies. This is now considered fraud. You either have to charge them like anyone else or do it all for free; it is all or nothing.

So here's what happens, not only are you concerned that you have to charge them, you also begin to worry about inconveniencing them as well. In urology, where often times a pelvic or rectal exam is necessary; this is thrown into the mix because you don't want to make someone feel uncomfortable. You might put off the exam for fear of embarrassing them.

If you decide to see them for free and determine they need an x-ray or blood work, then you now have to wade through how these tests will be paid. In addition, they ask as they are leaving an office visit this question, "Do I have to come back to get the results or can you just call me?" This not only is another thing you have to do without reimbursement it also puts you at risk by not completing the circle.

Now, you have broken several protective rules because you want to do right by a friend or relative, and you either have to pay for the tests you've ordered or broach that issue with them.

Lawyers have no qualms charging their friends, do they? Why do doctors feel we should be different? I have learned over time that the best way to treat friends, family and physicians is the same way you treat everyone. And guess what? They will get better care and you'll expose yourself to less risk.

Rule: Friends, family and fellow physicians get the worst care. In addition, if someone is going to have a complication, it will be a friend, family member, or fellow member of the medical community. You can take that to the bank. Or should I say the courthouse?

Corollary: "The doctor that treats himself has a fool for a patient."-Osler

78

I Ain't Saying I'm the Best - I'm Saying I'm Just as Good

My in-laws lived in Atlanta a while back and were visiting a friend in the hospital who had just had an open prostatectomy. During the visit, the patient told them that, "My surgeon said he does this surgery better than anyone in Atlanta. He said he helped develop the procedure."

My in-laws see me later that month and tell me about the visit with their friend and question me about the surgeon and what he had said.

"John do you know a urologist in Atlanta named Dr. Clayton Smith?"

"No I don't. I have never heard of him." I say.

In the old days, urologists did make a point of gathering at local meetings and it was not uncommon for all of the urologists of a state to be familiar with each other. When I came to Gainesville in 1986, the urologists here were members of the Atlanta Urological Society and as a result went to the meetings commonly and knew most of the Atlanta urologists. I, for better or worse, have never enjoyed the company of other urologists, particularly the ones that go to meetings. Barnyard roosters crowing about themselves insatiably come to mind and may be the reason I don't go to meetings anymore.

"He did a prostate surgery on a friend of ours and told him he was the best urologist in Atlanta. Can that be true? I mean can a person say that?"

"A person can say that but I think it would be hard prove or get any group of urologists to agree about it. He may have experience in that particular procedure but there a lot of urologists who do a prostatectomy well."

I continue, "If he did say that, it is probably a reflection of being new to the city and he that is trying to promote himself in a very competitive market. I think it would have been fairer for him to say, "I do this procedure as well as anyone.""

Rule: It is a sad dog that won't wag his own tail, but there are limits.

79
The Curse of Priapus

Priapus: a minor Greek fertility god best known for his large and permanently erect phallus. He was the son of Aphrodite and was cursed with impotence before birth by Hera. Priapus was a protector of gardens and orchards, and is typically portrayed as a homely old man with a raging erection.

Years ago, we had an endocrinologist in our community whose personality was such that his practice was not only small, but dwindling. He was not a bad guy, just odd. He falls into a common category of doctors you are likely to come across in your career. The doctor will call about a patient he has, and he wants advice regarding something a urologist does. It is not his intention to send you the patient; he wants to learn something. In this case, this doctor wanted to know how to treat diabetic-induced impotence with injection therapy. Oh yeah, he wanted to know all of my tricks: the size of the needle, where to put it, how to prescribe it, who compounded it in town, and also any complications related to the procedure. It starts with you being called away from your work to answer these questions, knowing that this guy is only probing for information and there is no way in hell a referral will come from it. I am sorry, but this has got to be nipped in the bud.

"If you are not careful with the dosing, priapism can occur. Although patients laugh when you tell them of this possibility, it is not a laughing matter. The corpora will need to be irrigated with a butterfly needle using a neosynephrine solution, and if that doesn't work, sometimes (and this gets them every time) a shunt is formed between the glans and the corpora using an eleven blade knife. It's a pretty bloody proposition. Certainly the possibility of impotence can occur if the erection lasts more than four hours and if the priapism is of the ischemic type." Silence follows. "Thank you," he says. "Maybe it would be better just to have you see this patient."

Rule: If you can't manage the complication of a procedure then don't do the procedure.

80
That's Two Years per Inch

Urologists get grief from everyone. It never ends; the innuendos, the slights, the veiled insults are perpetrated upon us from every direction. Our children's friends are brutal. "Your daddy works on penises."

I mean, you can be a board certified urologist and examining a young man who is concerned about contracting something at a bachelor's party, no less, and even here, even this guy, feels sorry for you and the profession you've chosen.

As I am checking to see if he caught anything, the young man says, "This must be a tough job having to do what you do." But before you think that urologists go into urology and put up with all this grief because it is easy (truth be told, it is) let us do the math, shall we?

Four years of college, four years of medical school and the five years of residency equals 13 years. Now, we do work on other areas of the genitourinary system but for now, to show you how complicated what we do is, for demonstration purposes I will limit my calculations to the penis.

The average penis (by urban legend) is 6 inches long; actually it is 5.6 inches or 14.2 cm. We'll use six for this demonstration.

So, 13 years divided by 6 equals 2.16 or approximately 2 years of study for each inch of penis. As you can see, the longer penises require less time of study-it's an inverse thing, and reinforces the notion of "it is not the length of the boat but the motion of the ocean."

Now this not only shows how complicated the penis is, I've not even started on the testicles and other stuff, but how dedicated urologists are in learning every inch of territory that is their trade.

Rule: Inch by inch life's, I mean urology, is a cinch. Urologists work below the belt and we know what small, medium and large is...my friend. Do not mess with us.

Man to wife: "Tell me something that will make me happy and sad at the same time." Wife to husband: "You have the biggest penis of all your friends."

81
You Chose Internal Medicine I Didn't

When I was the chief resident, one of the skills you needed was keeping your service clean. In other words, you can have a urology service in which the majority of the patients are non-surgical and replete with medical problems. On rounds everyone began to think, "What the hell is going on here? This looks like a medical service." Inheriting a dirty service by the outgoing chief resident is called being passed the shit baton. To a larger degree, the reverse is true for the internal medicine services. The chiefs of these services are trying to get anything surgical off their service and placed elsewhere.

"Hi, this is Dr. So and So in internal medicine. We have got this guy on our service that has swollen left testicle. He is stable medically and I hoping we could get him placed on urology. Would that be possible?"

"You mentioned that he was stable medically. What other 'stable' medical issues does this patient have?"

"Well, he has diabetes, hypertension, and vascular disease, but as I said, these issues are stable."

"I think from a urologic perspective, it would be best, in light of these stable issues, to have the patient remain on your service. I can take care of the scrotum without moving the patient."

"I have talked to my attending and he feels this patient should be on your service as it is clear that the pressing issue the scrotum."

"That's right, a scrotum surrounded by a shit load of other medical problems that will still be there when the scrotum is all better." You get the drift. This type of banter continues into private practice, but now it is not the internal medicine doctor, but the hospitalist; now it is a battle of who is the primary. I had little cards made up when I was chief of urology just for this type of situation. It read: You chose internal medicine, I didn't.

Rule: Why do you call internal medicine doctors fleas? Because they are the last thing to leave a dying dog.

82
I Don't See No...

A father and son are talking the night before the son is to be shipped off to sea in the Navy. The father, a Navy veteran, was telling the son some things to look out for on his extended trip on an aircraft carrier.

"Ed, now you know that you'll be on a ship with men for an extended period of time. There are some precautions that I want you to be aware of and be sure to be diligent about."

The father continued, "When you shower and someone drops their soap and asks you to pick it up, be sure to pick it up by not just bending over to get it. In other words, keep your knees together and squat as if you were a female with a dress on. You never know what men may be up to in these types of situations. Just be safe about it son."

After about two months on the ship, sure enough while taking a shower, someone drops their soap and asks Ed to pick it up and hand it to him. He remembers his father's admonition and does so by not bending over but by squatting with his knees together. This happens several times over the next ensuing weeks and each time he thwarts the perceived intention by his shipmates.

One day he is showering and across the way from him a sailor is looking out of a port hole and says, "Well would you look at that; a ship that has wheels!"
Ed goes to where the sailor is and bends over to look through the port hole to see the ship with wheels and says, "I don't see no wheeeeeeeeeeeeeeeeeeeeeeeeeeeeeeeeeealllls!"

Rule: No rule just a joke I heard in residency.

83

Do You Want It Too Short or Too Long?

I enjoyed the part of residency that involved working with interns and medical students who would rotate through urology, most of them, that is. If they were know-it-alls or had a chip on their shoulder, then I either made fun of them, excluded them from anything interesting, or ignored them. I never could get over a third year medical student questioning the wisdom regarding a urological issue posed by the chief resident, but it happened.

My favorite students were girls. The girls were fun to be with, smart, hardworking and had a better sense of humor than the men, who usually took themselves too seriously. There were several male surgical interns that rotated through that I had a ball with. One, an orthopedic intern, I taught how to do circumcisions on the prisoners of the ninth floor of Talmadge; apparently having to do a circumcision was a good change of pace for these patients. This intern and I became good friends. One day, we were in the urologic clinic and this orthopedic intern is reporting to me about a patient he has seen.

"The patient is a 65 year old male and he says he can't get but three erections a night. He is accustomed to having sex with younger females at his lake house, and relates he now can only have sex once." This pissed me off. As my mother would say, this guy had the "gall of eighty."

"You tell him that the treatment for his malady is abstinence for six months. We'll see the asshole back in the clinic at that time." What was funny was that the intern returns to the dictation area and dictates as a note exactly what he had told me and what I had told him to tell the patient. It was done perfectly and in a professional tone and voice. I often have wondered what the transcriptionist thought about that dictation.

Rule: If you are an intern or student, what is the perfect attitude to have with a senior resident? When asked to cut the suture, simply smile and say, "Too short or too long?" Just the right blend of humor admixed with a bit of "give it right back to 'em."

84
Is It Something You Can Live With?

This is a magical question for the urologist to ask the patient. I have had patients go on for minutes about a problem in great detail and how it has affected their lives. Then, after respectfully listening and taking notes for this issue, which is different than the problem the patient is there to see you for; they reveal that they don't want any treatment for it. It happens all the time and reinforces the belief that patients often just want to talk and share their problems with the doctor. Don't be frustrated when this happens, because you don't have to treat or recommend medicines for this compilation of symptoms. View what they have told you as a gift to do nothing. If the patient wants nothing, don't you go and do something. If you do, you are introducing a whole new set of variables that you may then have to manage. As the song by Arcade Fire says, "If you want something, don't ask for nothing. If you don't want nothing, don't ask for something." Or something like that, I guess, applies here.

So when the patient sits down, pulls out papers he printed from the internet and says, "May I ask you a few questions?" What is a urologist to do?

Well, you are stuck. You have to listen to all of them. Then you have to prioritize them and find out which "complaints" they can live with, and then deal with this amended list. Hopefully you can get to "What bothers you the most?" and move the office visit along. There is a skill to getting to what the patient feels is actionable, managing it and sending them on their way, content that their concerns were heard and addressed. This is what you must learn to master.

Rule: Listen first, but if it ain't broke, don't fix it.

Urologist: "Of all those symptoms, are any of them bad enough to take another medicine for?" Patient: "No."
There you have it!

85

Poor Planning On Your Part Doesn't Constitute an Emergency on Mine

This saying, as it applies both to patients and your physician colleagues, will come across as harsh and uncaring, but I feel its application is important for the new urologist to be aware.

A patient's wife calls your office on a Friday, fifteen minutes before closing time, and asks you to see her husband for kidney stone pain. After waiting minutes for the wife to find her husband and give the phone to him, he relates to the nurse, "The pain started a week ago and has been bad all day." The question then becomes do you see this patient and keep your staff late or recommend that this patient go to the emergency room? Does this aphorism apply? Hint: Don't forget the resultant aphorism consequence of obliging this patient and that is, "No good deed goes unpunished."

You tell the patient to come on and he says, after conferring with his wife, that he can be there in fifteen minutes. You negotiate with one of the members of your staff to stay late. The patient's son is going to miss dinner because of the stone and so demands to stop at McDonald's on the way. This pit stop in addition to dropping of the baby at momma's house results in the patient arriving an hour later. The pain and nausea is retractable to your IM injections and the wife wants him admitted to the hospital. It now has been two hours since the fateful phone call and now you begin the process of getting the patient admitted.

And then you remember that this has happened to you before and that you now have missed a family function. You vow not to let this happen again and wonder how you could have mismanaged your time and the patient so poorly.

If only you had simply said, "It would be in your best interest to go to the emergency room." He would have had an IV, all the medicines he needed, a definitive diagnosis with the CT scan the ER doctor would have done, completed lab values and the patient all teed up to be admitted with a phone call. Instead you have nothing but misplaced empathy that has wasted two hours of yours and the patient's time.

Rule: "Begin with the end in mind." *The Seven Habits of Highly Successful People*

Plan your work; work your plan.
Fail to plan; plan to fail.

"Even if you are on the right track, you'll get run over if you just sit there."-Will Rogers

86
The Mind of an Anesthesiologist-Part 1

One of my oldest friends in my town is an anesthesiologist. I met him on the burn service at Talmadge when I was an intern and he was a senior medical student. On that service was a patient who had been doused with gas while shaving and set on fire by a scorned lover. This patient needed subclavian lines changed several times a week and, ironically, I taught my friend how to do central lines. This is something I remind him of in front of his associates on a regular basis. As you know, the relationship between the anesthesiologist and the surgeon is often adversarial in nature. My being friends with this guy, however, has allowed me to have a more compassionate view of our anesthesiologist colleagues. Always remember, they want to be doctors too.

This "gas passer" and I have the best time pretending we hate each other and each other's specialty in front of the operating room staff. We are kidding, but if you didn't know that, you would think that we were being very rude to each other. The following is one such exchange.

I am doing a sling and sitting between the legs of a lady in the pelvic position. My friend the anesthesiologist enters the room and begins to talk to the anesthetist.

I look up and say angrily, "Could you please be quite Dr. Winham, I am working on the human vagina here!" Uncharacteristically my friend adopts an apologetic tone.

"Dr. McHugh, I am so sorry. How could I have been so inconsiderate?"

Then addressing the room he says, "Everyone, you have to understand. This is the closest Dr. McHugh has been to a vagina in six months!"

That was a good comeback. It left me silent and at a loss for words. He was on his game that day, which is unusual.

Rule: Damn it! I forgot he knew I'd had my prostate removed. Truth hurts.

87
Dr. Winham, I Am Limiting My Practice to Only Large Penises

W e were doing a urology review during my residency and somewhere in the article the author says that the urologist is the natural choice for a man to speak to about impotence. His reasoning was that urologists are earthy people. I'd add thick skinned to that.

How many times have you been with other physicians or with a group of people, and it comes up that you are a urologist. "How do you do that all day?" This is a benign enough remark, but with time and maybe alcohol the jibes become a bit more piercing and, worse yet, personal. As a urologist you have to see this type of situation and nip it in the bud. Here's how you do it.

So Winham says to me in front of a group of other men, "John, why do men go into urology? Is it because they like..."

Here's where you cleverly intervene.

"Hey I have an announcement to make. As my patient volume has grown, I have decided to limit my practice."

"Really?"

"Yes. From now on I am limiting my practice to only large penises."

I continue, "Winham, you will be getting a letter from my office soon. I will no longer be able to see you as a patient."

Rule: Never mess with a urologist especially if you have seen him as a patient. At any time he may play the penis card.

Dr. Winham: "Dr. McHugh you are a poor surgeon and you only bring sick patients with a myriad of underlying health problems to the hospital and expect me to keep them alive long enough for you to work on."
Dr. McHugh: "Dr. Winham, you have a small penis that not only works sporadically, but when it does, it works too quickly satisfying no one else but yourself."
Silence...
Exactly what the urologist hoped to achieve.

88
People, Events and Ideas

"Great minds discuss ideas; average minds events; and small minds people."
Eleanor Roosevelt.

My mother was in the Coast Guard during World War II and loved F.D.R.; she particularly loved Eleanor Roosevelt. She was a lifelong democrat just like everyone else who was alive during that era.

But about this quote: in many ways it is a reflection of what one might hear physicians talking about in the doctor's dining room or the surgeon's lounge. The problem is, however, that the subject matter you'll overhear will be of the small mind type and maybe a smidgen of the average.

Here are some common topics of discussion:

- Medicare doesn't pay enough.
- Insurance's don't pay enough.
- Anesthesia (not a doctor have you) cancelled my case.
- The hospital EMR sucks/the hospital sucks.
- Looking at the OR schedule and discussing it.
- The milk in the refrigerator is old.
- What they did while on call/who came in the ER.
- A little smattering of sports talk
- What is the menu in the dining room today
- Bitching about turnover time in OR

My brother-in-law had a bumper sticker on his car that read: "I hate people and most insects." I might add doctors to that. Or how about this one: I used to be a people person, but people ruined it for me.

Rule: If you want to have an interesting conversation with someone, then you might want to steer clear of the medical profession. Events and people will dominate the affair.
"While medicine is to be your vocation, or calling, see to it that you have also an avocation-some intellectual pastime which may serve to keep you in touch with the world of art, of science, or of letters."-Osler

89
The Surgeon's Finest Hour

The surgeon's finest hour? Well of course it is draining pus; this is one of the oldest of all aphorisms, right up there with "A chance to cut is a chance to cure."

What would you say is the urologist's finest hour? Take any elective surgical procedure off the table (no pun intended). What do you think in private practice will be your most frequent consultation?

You see, in private practice when patients present to the emergency room with a urological problem and significant other medical issues, the hospitalist admits, and you are the consultant. If a CT scan has been done and there is the dreaded combination of an obstruction and azotemia, then you as the urologist are stuck with two dilemmas. And by the way, these dilemmas will occur at the most inconvenient time for you and your schedule.

Dilemma one: You decide that the patient is too sick to place a stent under anesthesia. You then make the brilliant deduction that you will call the interventional radiologist to place a nephrostomy. The interventional radiologist will have a series of questions for you. The first: "Is this necessary?" and you will have to refrain yourself from descending into combative sarcasm. The second: "Did you know there is an element of risk in putting a needle into the kidney and bleeding?" If you want to subject yourself to this line of questioning have at it.

Dilemma two: You choose the lesser of two evils, and you schedule a stent placement, letting the anesthesiologist deal with the medical issues. If, by chance, he demurs, it is not the end of the world. Your hands are tied; you call the I.R. guy back with your new ammunition for a nephrostomy. You are not treating a patient with a stone; you are treating a stone that happens to have a patient. That is what anesthesia is for.

Rule: Nature is a good physician but a poor surgeon.

90
James Brown's Father

This story is about 95% true and has to do with a patient of mine when I was a junior urology resident at the VA in Augusta, Georgia.

I go into a room in the urology clinic and there is an older man in wheelchair there, who as I recall, was named James Brown Sr. I pretty sure he was a senior because otherwise I would not have made the connection. I knew that James Brown had a home in Augusta and that he was raised across the Savannah River in Beach Island, South Carolina.

"Are you *the* James Brown's father?"

"Yes, I am."

What I said next I don't know why I said it. It may be because I was curious as to why he was getting his medical care in a VA versus having a personal physician.

"Do you see James Brown much?"

"My son treats me just fine, thank you," he said a bit curtly.

Mr. Brown had a hydrocele. This was repaired the following week. I had just seen him and was leaving the nurses' station when a nurse said there was a call for me. It was James Brown inquiring as to the condition of his father.

"How is my father?" he asked.

"Mr. Brown, everything went just fine. Your papa's got a brand new bag! "

At the twenty-year LaGrange High School Reunion Class of 73, I was awarded "graduate with most interesting job." Upon accepting my "award" and at the behest of my "friends" I told the above story.

Rule: James Brown had prostate cancer in 2004 and was treated in Atlanta, Georgia.

Hugh Hampton Young was studying bladder dysfunction under Dr. James Brown at Johns Hopkins until Brown died suddenly. Subsequently, the position of the dispensary of genitourinary diseases was given to Young by William Halsted in 1897. Young was 27 and for over forty years was the head of the department of urology.

91

The Difficult We Handle Immediately-The Impossible Takes a Little Longer

There is a contemporary of mine when I started in Gainesville who was a pulmonologist. As was common at that time, the pulmonologist served as the hospital's intensivist. In private practice it is unusual for the urologist to have patients in intensive care, and if there is one in this unit, the urologist is a duck out of water. If a urologist's patient is in there it is commonly associated with a procedure he has performed. So for many reasons, it is an unpleasant and bad sign if you have a patient in ICU.

You go into the room with all the monitors going, pressors and antibiotics are hanging everywhere; all is unfamiliar. All you can muster to the nurse is, "The urine in the foley looks clear. Has Dr. Murray been by?"

When I found myself in need of Dr. Murray's services, before I'd call I'd prepare my spiel and make sure I knew all the medicines, surgeries, allergies and heart history of the patient; I wanted my guns loaded for the barrage of questioned I knew would result from my call for help. I'd rationalize that this patient's need of an ICU bed was not my fault; I did the surgery to help. I'm the good guy, right? "Tom, this is John McHugh. May I tell you about a patient I'd like you to see for me?"

"Sure John, whatcha got?"

"A fifty-five year old male, in whom I removed a stone endoscopically, is in the recovery room and anesthesia cannot maintain his pressure and his oxygen saturation is not good. I..." At that Tom, God bless his soul, interrupts me and says, "John, do you need me to make him all better?"

"Please," I say.

"I'll take care of it. What's his name and where is he?"

Rule: Urology is a specialty: if someone calls for help, even if they have mucked up the urethra trying to put in a catheter and blood is everywhere, just help them and leave off the theatrics.
Don't celebrate in the end zone after a touchdown. Act like you've been there before.

92

You Can Mess With a Man's Wife but You'd Better Not Mess with His Livelihood

Okay, this one I just remember hearing. It is really more about how important it is to a male about being the bread winner than whether that is more important than his wife. It makes the point that men in general, and surgeons in particular, are territorial— both in protecting their referral pattern, but also the procedures they perform. You probably take performing the transobturator sling for granted don't you? Well, other than this procedure, how often do you make a vaginal incision? Hmmmmmm?

There was a gynecologist who I worked with often, and over time we developed a relationship regarding surgeries that were unusual for that time. If he had a patient who needed an AP repair and had stress incontinence, he'd ask me to do the sling. But we did things differently than was the norm for surgeons at that time. He would make a vaginal incision and correct the cystocele, and then he'd make the posterior incision for the rectocele, repair it, and then close it, leaving the anterior incision open. I would enter the room, he'd leave, I'd do the sling (at that time it was the cadaver sling that was used and was attached to the pubic bone by way of screws that were drilled into place. Weird, huh?), and then I'd close the anterior vaginal incision. This sounds straightforward and simple, doesn't it? However, at this time the idea of making an incision that you don't stay around to close was unheard of. It all started with me saying to this gynecologist, "You can stay to close your incision, but I am here and I can do it. You can go have coffee or something." It was revolutionary for the time and did not go unnoticed by competing gynecologists in our community, particularly the older more predatory ones.

One day I am beginning to place a sling and I have the feeling that someone is behind me. I turn and it is a gynecologist moving into my space and peering into the vagina, the same one who told a patient of mine I couldn't make a straight incision because I was young.

"You know John, the vagina is very vascular. It will bleed on ya if you don't know what you're doing."

I as sarcastically a tone as I could conjure up I reply, "Thank you so much. Seeing as how I have only done about two hundred of these, I'll keep that in mind. You are in my light, if you don't mind."

Rule: I'd wager that the penis is just as vascular as the vagina and "harder" to work on. I do have to admit however, they both are tough; so tough that a dog can't bite it and a cat can't scratch it!

"In life's perspective we seniors are apt to resent that the rising generation should work out its own salvation in ways that are not always our ways, and with thoughts that are not always our thoughts."-Osler

93
Three Types of Lies- Lies, Damned Lies and Statistics

*I*f all you have is a hammer then the whole world is a nail. I am sure a lot of good comes out of tumor conferences: doctors gathered of different specialties lending their expertise to do what is best for the patient, or at least that is the intended goal. I was a member of the tumor committee for several years and went to many meetings. When I learned about how things played out as it pertains to prostate cancer and the discussions this disease prompted I quit going to them.

Tumor committees usually have an oncologist and, of course, in those cases where chemotherapy had a role an oncologist will generally recommended chemotherapy. This, in turn, prompts a recitation of studies by the radiation therapist showing that radiation either alone or in combination with chemotherapy yielded the best results. The same debate would then ensue over and over each month with each side promoting his specialty.

Now if the discussion were prostate cancer, the oncologist did not have "a dog in that fight," so the competition then became between the radiation therapist and the urologist. I did not play along with this gamesmanship; but I did enjoy when other urologists attended the meeting, and I could watch the surgery vs. radiation debate.

"The studies show that regardless of the treatment method, the fifteen-year survival rate is the same. With radiation, the risks of bleeding, impotence and incontinence are much less and etc. etc." Anyone can find a study or statistic to support a viewpoint. Also, radiation therapists have never met a prostate cancer they didn't like. This is true for the urologist as well; the "a chance to cut is a chance to cure" mentality pervades their mindset as well.

Rule: As much as doctors like to tout this or that study, why not give patients an honest appraisal of the options and let them decide? *Supporting studies tend to "paint the bull's eye around the well placed arrow."*

94
Revenge is a Desert Best Served Cold

"Patience is bitter, but its fruit is sweet."
Jean-Jacques Rousseau

W hen I started my career, the only reliable procedure for stress incontinence was an MMK procedure. They had slings back in those days but you had to harvest the fascia from the thigh area and then it was guess work as to how tight to make it. As a result, few people did those types of procedures; I witnessed the harvesting by an older gynecologist and it was barbaric.

I usually did the MMK with my partner, however, from time to time I'd be asked to do it in conjunction with the gynecologist after he'd done a hysterectomy. It was a nice arrangement and in time I was able to negotiate that the gynecologist would make the incision and remove the uterus. Then I would come in to do the MMK and close the incision.

I was asked to do a MMK with a lady using the above scenario but the older partner, of whom I never worked with, was scheduled to do the procedure. In addition, it was not for a hysterectomy, but for an oophorectomy, and I was told to go first instead of my usual second. At the time of my Pfannenstiel incision, I noted that she has had a previous incision there. I decide to excise the old scar and make the superior portion of the elliptical incision with the intention of doing the lower half at the end of the procedure. That's right; I was not to be there at the end; my routine had been disrupted. I do the MMK and leave, they call the GYN and he completes the procedure. I forgot about the lower half of the incision.

The next day, upon seeing the patient she says, "Dr. McHugh, I asked Dr. So and So why my incision was crooked. He said that you were new and didn't know how to make a straight incision. Is that true?" It dawned on me what had happened and I explained it to her and apologized for it. It, however, was not lost on me that this doctor could have easily noted the scar and excised it. To him it was an opportunity.

The next day on rounds she says, "Dr. McHugh, today the other doctor said that urologists have no business working on the bladder and doing the procedure you did on me. Is that true?" Still giving this doctor the benefit of the doubt, I explain that both GYNs and urologists do the procedure and assured her that urologists did bladder work all the time.

On the third day, the subversive actions of this "colleague" continued. My patient says, "Dr. McHugh, today he wanted to know what doctor had referred me to you. That my family doctor had done a disservice in sending patients with my problem to a urologist, particularly ones that didn't know what they doing." After a pause she added, "Why is he doing this to you?"

This was my first encounter with someone practicing old-fashioned "turf protection" in an unethical fashion. I noted it and never forgot it. This patient saw through what he was attempting to do, and she even felt sorry for the guy. I have since seen her husband and her over the last twenty five years and consider her one of my many patient friends.

Rule: So many rules...let's see: Burn me once shame on you, burn me twice shame on me. Just as parents know their kids, and wives their husbands, so too patients know the person behind the doctor. Patients are smarter and more observant than most doctors give them credit for. And what did Dr. Witherington tell me? "He'll need your help one day."

"Never believe what a patient tells you his doctor has said."-William Jenner

Corollary: "Be suspicious of what a doctor tells a patient about another doctor or you." As my mother said, "consider the source."

"If you can't say anything good about a man, say nothing."-Osler

95
New Dress, Same Whore

It has been slow in coming, but I feel that the robotic prostatectomy has considerable advantages over the open prostatectomy. I might add the caveat that this is true only for the surgeon who can do one well. The benefits are an almost guaranteed one night hospital stay, a better anastomosis with the resultant less catheter time, acceptable operative time, less blood loss, and, of course, the fact that seven small incisions heal quicker and with less pain than one four inch incision. Again, there is no argument from me on these points if performed by someone who has done a bunch of robotic procedures and has a knack for it.

Oh, wait a minute. What about the things that really count? You remember, don't you, the trifecta: cure, potency and continence? If these are not achieved, have the same incidence as an open prostatectomy, and are performed the wrong person, then the robotic method is nothing more than a new dress on the same whore. No matter how it is done, you are still removing the prostate and putting things back together with the same potential deleterious consequences.

And by the way, I am okay with the robotic method; I had my prostate removed that way. I do take issue with urologists not giving their patients the whole story on the procedure's results, and their performing it as it pertains to cure, potency and continence.

Two weeks after a robotic prostatectomy, a patient tells a friend, "It was great. Went home in a day, and I am already walking around and driving." What you don't hear is that little angel (or urologic devil) on the patient's shoulder asking, "What did your path report show? Are you having erections? And why don't you tell him about how it feels to be wearing a diaper?"

My mother often said to me, "To thine own self be true." I might add to this, "To thine patients be true."

I know, I know. The guy that has done five hundred had to hone his skill on the first fifty. I don't know what else to tell you other than what Lou Holtz told his players at Notre Dame: "Do right."

Rule: I have to use this one again; it is perfect for the urologist's use of the robot. "A fool with a tool is still a fool."

"Let man learn to be honest and do the right thing or do nothing."
-James Marion Sims

Patient to urologist: "Vasectomies don't take very long to do. Are they easy to perform?"
Urologist: "After the first five hundred they are."

This is true of every procedure that is performed and appears easy.

96
Rearranging the Chairs on the Titanic

One day, what I am about to describe will happen to you and you will remember what you read here. I have often said, "If it has happened to me, or if I have thought of it, then it has happened, or is going to happen, to someone else." This is one of those things.

The patient you are presented with is an eighty year old lady who has numerous medical problems. After having been admitted for "the dwindles," it becomes known that there is bilateral lower ureteral obstruction by a pelvic malignancy and a creatinine of four. You are consulted to unblock the obstruction.

When you enter the room, the patient's extended family is there and everyone has the countenance of grave concern. After introducing yourself, you explain that there are three major options from your perspective. One is to divert the urine by way of bilateral stents. Option two is to divert with nephrostomies. And, option three is to do nothing.

You explain that even if the kidney function is corrected, then the patient still has the pelvic malignancy, for which the prognosis in and of itself is not curative and will most likely result in the patient's demise.

It is here that someone in the room needs to be a big boy. On the emotional side of things, the family will initially want to "do everything possible for mamma." The easy thing for you to do is simply be a technician, put in the stents, move along and leave the remaining medical problems to the family and the other specialists.

Or, you could initiate the hard discussion that further intervention is only putting off the inevitable. Here's the thing, dying of uremia is a fairly nice way to die. Ureteral obstruction and azotemia is a gift in some situations. Do you want to correct the creatinine, only to have the patient then suffer with the consequences of the pelvic malignancy? You have to help the family see beyond the current crisis. In my opinion, at least broach the subject; one of the family members may get the picture. We pursued this line of inaction when my grandmother was in this situation. She died in her bed in her home without tubes and in peace. It was a beautiful thing to behold.

Rule: Help the family see how things play out with scenarios of doing something vs. doing nothing. It may surprise you how smart a family can be. The reverse is true as well.

"The value of experience is not in seeing much, but in seeing wisely."-Osler

97
Best Way to Double Your Money

D o you know anyone who has been taken in by a Ponzi scheme? I do: me. As they say, "A word to the wise is sufficient." As it pertains to investing, let me tell you, "Experience is a great teacher. It has helped me recognize my mistakes the second time I make them."

A doctor friend of mine told me of an investment he was doing along with several other doctors and people in town that I knew and respected professionally. I ended up participating and initially it all went swimmingly, but in time it became clear that we were in a shell game and when one of the major investors needed to cash out, the money wasn't there for other investors following suit, and the whole scheme came tumbling down. Ironically, this was about the time of the Madoff scandal in New York, and, as a result, congress enacted favorable tax benefits for those unfortunate souls who had fallen for Ponzi schemes. This softened the blow. But, in retrospect, the whole affair epitomized the saying: "If it is too good to be true, then it probably is." It also manifested one of the deadliest of the seven deadly sins: greed. But, I learned my lesson and moved on. Well, I did move on but it was a tough time, very tough. Remember what Rudyard Kipling said about finding yourself in a situation like this in "If."

> *If you can make one heap of all your winnings*
> *And risk it on one turn of pitch-and-toss,*
> *And lose, and start again at your beginnings*
> *And never breath a word about your loss;*

My advice is diversified mutual funds and dollar cost averaging starting right now. Saving is not doing without; it is paying yourself first.

Rule: The best way to "double your money" is to fold it in half and put it back in your pocket.

"Laugh hard. It's a long way to the bank." "Paper Thin Walls" by Modest Mouse

98

Never Say "He's Bucking" to an Anesthesiologist

I have the highest respect for the specialty of **anus**thesia. I'm sorry, did I misspell that? I meant to say anesthesia. It helps that the most senior anesthesiologist at our hospital and I did a burn unit rotation in the early eighties. I taught him how to start a central line. I enjoy our banter about the conflicting and constantly clashing attributes of the surgeon and the anesthesiologist. He does not mince words when it comes to patient care or putting a surgeon in his place.

"John, I am either going to hammer you down to nothing with logic, emphasizing how wrong you are, or I will make a fool of you, highlighting your ignorance. It is your choice."

So Dr. Winham is the anesthesiologist at my group's surgery center, and I have a student tech with me one day. I am doing a hydrocele and the patient begins to move. The student is about to say something to Dr. Winham, and I stop her.

I say, "It looks like he is not paying attention to the patient and that he is just checking the email on his phone; nothing could be further from the truth. He is in tune with this patient and will correct this lapse in anesthesia at a time of his choosing. Do not, I repeat, do not tell him that this patient is "bucking." Anesthesiologists in general and this one in particular don't take well to the word "bucking."

I continue, "You have to do and say subtle things that he might overhear or notice; this way, correcting things is his idea. I, for one, am not going to tell Dr. Winham that the patient is waking up."

The student, who was forty and had been an executive in a previous life then asks, "What if he doesn't notice, can I tell him then?"

I say, "Let's ask him. Dr. Winham, the student wants to know at what point it would be appropriate for her to tell you that the anesthesia is getting light and that the patient is moving."

Dr. Winham ponders for a second and says, "Never. You don't speak to me. If anyone speaks to me, it should be the surgeon. Even then, I don't tell him what suture to use, and he ain't telling me how to do anesthesia."

Rule: Here's the thing: anesthesiologists think they are doctors too and would have been surgeons if they had had the hands for it. Just play along.

"What is the student but a lover courting a fickle mistress who ever eludes his grasp?"-Osler

A physician is someone who knows everything and does nothing.
A surgeon is someone who does everything and knows nothing.
A urologist is someone who works on the "little head" not the "big head," and advises young men not to think with the "wrong head."
An anesthesiologist is someone half asleep keeping a patient half awake.
A psychiatrist is someone who knows nothing and does nothing.
A pathologist is someone who knows everything and does everything too late.

Urology: It ain't rocket surgery and it ain't brain science.

There once was a urologist from Bambini
Who spilt some gin on his wennie
Not to be uncouth
He spilt some vermouth
And slipped his date a Martini

Definition of a cystoscope: An instrument with a prick at both ends.

99
You're Not Leaving My Office Without One

I currently have as a patient a ninety plus year old man who has thirteen children and over a hundred grandchildren of various "great" descriptions. He always comes to the office with the eleventh child, a daughter, and wearing overalls.

"Do you know all their names, Mr. King?"

"No, but I think I have met them all."

Several years ago, I spent an afternoon in Wal-Mart buying all the accoutrements of one of my overhauls. This consisted of a watch, a chain, a clip for the watch chain (there's a hole for it), a wallet, a knife, and, finally, a carpenters pencil. I had to go to Home Depot for the pencil, and the all the ones they had were bright orange and had their name on it. I bought twenty. I looked online for a carpenter pencil you could put your company name on...no luck. You can do that with regular pencils, but not carpenter pencils.

So, one day Mr. King and number eleven are in the office. "I have something for you," I say.

I go and get one of the pencils and then put it in the slot of the overalls that is made for a carpenter pencil. I tried to shave it to expose the lead but just messed it up and made a mess in the exam room.

The last several visits to office he has conveniently forgotten to "wear" his pencil. This necessitates me having to go back to my office to get him another one.

"You are not leaving my office without a pencil Mr. King," I say.

Rule: You come into my office in overalls; you ain't leaving without a carpenter pencil for the pocket that was made for it. Always give 'em a little more than they paid for.

"Be charitable before wealth makes thee covetous."-Sir Thomas Browne

100
"Vincent, How Do You Do It Day after Day?"

I have a patient who is 89 and has a hundred or so patents. Every time I see him in the office, he tells me he is actively working on another. I told him about this book, and how I hoped to give him one at his next visit in six months. When I told him it was about sayings and aphorisms, he was fascinated. He became animated, said he'd love to have one and then that he had a story for me.

"Years ago, I was working with a famous heart surgeon at Johns Hopkins. I was working on an artificial heart valve, and this surgeon was helping me with the clinical aspects of the device. One day, I was with him in a Hopkins surgery observation theater when a resident yelled up to him that the bleeding would not stop. Vincent yelled back down to them to just "put a stitch in it" and close the patient, which the team did and the patient was taken to the recovery room."

Vincent said, "Day after day Ival, patients with bad problems come in here with difficult diseases that we may or may not be able to help. Many will have the surgery, we'll close them and they'll die in the recovery room. We then will be faced with the same situation tomorrow and into the foreseeable future; day in and day out. "

"Vincent, how do you do this every day? How do you continue doing surgery that may or may not help and then see all of your efforts done in vain and result in death?"

Vincent said to me, "Ival, you have to have a bad memory."

Rule: W.C. Fields, as was his custom, came home late and drunk. His wife angrily accosted him and said, "W.C. I hope you one day die in a vat of whiskey!" He replied, "Death in a vat of whiskey? Death where is thy sting?"

"Though it be in the power of the weakest arm to take away life, it is not in the strongest to deprive us from death."-Sir Thomas Browne

101
The Mind of an Anesthesiologist Part 2-
Winhamisms

Winham: "If you wanted a still field, then you should have gone into pathology."

McHugh: "I am so sorry, Dr. Winham. I told this patient that he wouldn't be feeling anything."

Winham: "I did not say I was cancelling your case; I said I was not providing anesthesia for it."

McHugh: "Dr. Winham can you hear the patient groaning in pain? What are you providing, *vocal* anesthesia?"

Winham: "Why is it that when the surgeon is slow it is because the case is difficult, but when the surgery is delayed by a difficult intubation it is the anesthesiologist's fault?"

McHugh: "Dr. Winham may have a small penis but it is not very big around." Dr. Winham's reply: "At least mine works."

Winham: "However long a surgeon tells you a case will take, triple it. The inverse is true if he is talking about the size of his penis."

McHugh: "Dr. Winham has a mirror above his bedroom bed that reads: Objects in mirror are larger than they appear. "

Winham: Dr. Winham, reviewing the parameters of the O.R. monitors and heart rhythm with a colleague says, "Dr. McHugh, don't mind us. It's just doctor talk."

McHugh: "Dr. Winham, a patient whom you've intubated brought in another tooth today to the office. Do you want it or shall I put it in a denture cup with the other teeth of patients of yours?"

McHugh: "Dr. Winham, *your* patient is moving!

Winham: "Oh really? Why don't you quit hurting him?"

McHugh: "Dr. Winham, this patient has moved the entire procedure and now it's taking you thirty minutes to wake him up. Where did you learn that technique? The sleep number mattress school? Winham, you and your kind are simply parasites, that's right, it is not even symbiosis. You are nothing without me. I feed you! I bring you cases and all I get from you is bitching about their weight, their medicines, that their blood pressure is high and comments about where in the hell did I find them. How about a thank-you for a change? ”

Winham: “Dr. McHugh, I am cancelling your case, thank-you.”

McHugh: “Why, for what reason?”

Winham: “Dr. McHugh, I can explain it to you, but I can't understand it for you!”

McHugh: “I want a different anesthesiologist. Why do I always get stuck with your sorry ass?”

Winham: “We were making assignments and your name came up. We drew straws and I lost.”

So Dr. Winham has been working on a prototype for the Winham Anesthesia NPO App; the issue of NPO status and the anesthesiologist's appraisal of this comes up commonly in the pre-operative area. The way the App works is that you plug in the variables of what the patient ate or drank and it figures out how long the patient, and the surgeon, have to wait to have the "anesthesia clearance" to proceed.

One day in our surgery center I was posing to Dr. Winham various scenarios and how the App might work.

"Dr. Winham. My patient has had one tsp of grits and one sip of coffee. How long do we have to wait until he can have his surgery?"

"Did the coffee have cream or was it black? The grits, instant or regular? How old is he and how much does he weigh?"

"Black and instant. He's fifty and two hundred pounds."

He then pretends to plug into his iPhone all of the facts of the NPO breaches and after a period of time says, "Eight hours."

"Can I try another scenario please?"

"Sure," Winham says, "what ya got?"

"My patient has had one fourth of a cup of orange juice and one small bite of a biscuit but he didn't swallow it."

"Did the biscuit have butter? Was the orange juice pulp or pulp free? Where was the biscuit cooked?"

"No butter, pulp free and McDonald's."

"Eight hours," is his answer and it is completely unapologetic in tone. He and his App are so smug. He doesn't even think twice about inconveniencing the surgeon under the guise of protecting the patient. He so wishes he were a urologist.

Always Give Them a Little More than They Paid For

From *The Decision*

When my children were young, I purchased several hundred dollars' worth of magic tricks in which the success of the trick was based more on its cost than my skill as a magician. The more I spent on the trick, the easier it was to perform and the more it appeared as magic. I had about 30 of them, and my favorite was a handkerchief that had a bra hidden inside.

To perform the trick you ask a woman, usually the teacher of my particular child at the time, to place the middle part of the handkerchief into the front of her blouse or shirt. I would place a student on each side of the teacher with each holding an opposite end of the handkerchief. After saying "abra cadabra," I would instruct them to pull each end. This resulted in the middle part popping out as a bra. I would very quickly gather up the bra and handkerchief and exclaim, "Oh my goodness, I am so sorry."

It was a big hit every time I did it, and, of course, the trick cost a lot. On one occasion, after I'd performed the trick for my son Sam's second grade class, a grandmother of one of the students approached me at a PTA function: "John, my grandson told me something very interesting this afternoon. He said, 'Grandma, you should have been in my class today. Dr. McHugh did a trick and took Ms. Wolfe's panties off!'"

Something else interesting occurred after the bra trick in Ms. Wolfe's classroom that day. As I was gathering up my magic tricks, she approached me and whispered into my ear, "John, what makes that trick so remarkable is that I haven't worn a bra since the seventies."

A patient of mine who had prostate cancer and whose prostate I had removed told me one day during a visit that he was a clown, but he could not do tricks. I told him about my little show, and over the next few years I did several events with him where he'd do the clowning and I'd do the tricks. As a gift, he gave me an excellent clown book on making balloon animals.

Before each example of an animal there would be a saying; I remember one distinctly. "Always give 'em a little more than they paid for." This saying has served me well over the years as a surgeon. My clown friend passed away several years later due to lung disease that resulted from his inhaling cement dust during a mission trip. He died with a clown figurine dangling from the ceiling above his bed in his hospital room. So, here you go, what follows is "a little more than you paid for," in honor of a clown who was both a patient and a friend.

John McHugh

"The arrival of a good clown exercises a more beneficial influence upon the health of a town than twenty asses laden with drugs."-Sydenham

102

"It's Smaller Now Doc than before You Worked on Me!"

Just as you have to be patient in recommending surgery for ED and prostatism, so too should you proceed with caution in the surgical management of Peyronies disease. Think of neurosurgeons recommending back surgery; it is the same concept.

If you have elected to remove a plague, then what if you damage the dorsal nerve and now the patient has a straight penis with no feeling? Or worse yet, because of your efforts, the penis has lost its ability to tumesce and it is still crooked. Do you think you'll live that one down? That's a real practice builder alright.

But I want to speak about doing a plication, which is what I prefer to do for Peyronies. As you know, before any surgical recommendation you need to wait six months to a year to let the Peyronies run its course. During this time, you can throw some Vitamin E at it or punish the patient for having the disease by prescribing Potaba. (That's four .5gm tablets six times a day. Talk about a compliance buster!) Or, how does injecting Verapamil directly into the plague sound to you if you were the patient? Have you ever seen the ecchymosis that results from the injection therapy? It is brutal and must be repeated several times.

So, the patient has tried the conservative measures for Peyronies, and you've elected to recommend a Peyronies plication for the curvature. You explain to the patient that the plication takes up the slack on the opposite of the plaque and will straighten the penis, but at the expense of length. I draw this out on exam room paper. I show the curve, where the stitches will be and how the length will shorten based on the degree of curvature; the more the curvature, the more the penis length will shorten. Despite this, the patient will always negate the straight penis he has and emphasize the loss of length. This is why, even though it doesn't help the patient remember, I always say that the plication is the last resort.

In other words, you must ask: "You are unable have suitable sex with the current curvature of your penis. Is that correct?"

Postoperatively: "Damn doc, it's straight but you took off three inches. You didn't leave me anything!"

Rule: Men will never tell the urologist, "It was shorter before you worked on me." It's not in their DNA.

As they say, "One inch more a King, one inch less a Queen."

103
Hair on the Chin- Difficult Intubation/ A Small Scrotum with Thick Rugae- Difficult Vasectomy

Did you know that red headed patients are a little bit more difficult to administer anesthesia? People who have had a recent weight gain and have a short neck are more likely to have sleep apnea. For the anesthesiologist, a history of a difficult intubation is something to take note of and something to take precautions for in advance of the attempt at intubation.

Did you know that men with certain features about their face they don't like are more likely to have a moustache? What do you think an anesthesiologist thinks when he sees a red headed guy with a goatee? Well he thinks that the guy has a goatee because he has a "weak chin" and he knows that a weak chin means that the trachea has anatomical characteristics that will make the intubation more difficult. Over time and as a specialist you begin to notice these things, and the "noticing" makes one a better doctor and allows for preparing for something that might go awry.

Anesthesiologists have no place to stand if, in an elective case, the patient has had something to eat, and he allows the case to proceed. If the patient aspirates and endures all that that entails and the anesthesiologist knew about it ahead of time; well, he is the proverbial "toast."

In urology, as time goes by you too will begin to notice characteristics about your patient that will give you a heads up. The heads up may make you decide to do a procedure at the hospital vs. your office or surgery center.

There are a many examples of this in urology but the first that comes to mind is in regards to doing a vasectomy. First of all, it is a procedure usually done in the office, through a small incision with local anesthesia and maybe a bit of oral pre-medication.

What if, in addition to those limitations, the patient is slightly rotund, has a small scrotum with thick skin and rugae?

What if he tells you he doesn't do well at the dentist, faints at the sight of blood and needles, and that lidocaine has no effect on him?

Every urologist has a vasectomy disaster story, and proceeding ahead to do a vasectomy in the above scenario increases the chances of it happening to you.

Rule: The slick surgeon's cases go well often times because of their penchant for patient selection.

Ureteroscopically, a mid-ureteral stone in a male with a big prostate is infinitely more difficult to do than a distal ureteral stone in a female. If you planned your treatment strategy accordingly, would not that make your "scheme" more easily achievable? Maybe the former should have lithotripsy or vine ripened a bit to allow for it to move distally, and the latter allowed to pass or plucked forthwith.

"When schemes are laid in advance, it is surprising how often the circumstances fit in with them."-Osler

104
If the Ureter Gives you Something Keep it

Have you ever noticed that when you begin to pass a stent over a glide wire that the scrub nurse will try to help by pushing the stent until they see the glide wire exit the distal end of the stent and then holding the glide wire at the end, push the stent toward the bladder? You got to watch them because what they invariably do is push the stent in with one hand and pull the glide wire with the other, pulling the glide wire out.

If the area you worked so hard to bypass is proximal, it is possible that this maneuver will bring the wire just distal to that area and as a result you have lost access. You may figure it out with fluoroscopy, or you may figure it out when you determine that he stent meets resistance and won't go into the renal pelvis and, worse yet, your attempts to do so now have made it harder to replace the wire where you had it. What a mess.

If you are a urologist, then this has happened to you. How about this one: after having placed a wire past a tricky area, and you are sliding the stent over the wire, unbeknownst to you, the nurse begins using the pusher to advance the stent, resulting in the wire looping into the bladder. This premature maneuver on the part of your "helper" results in redundant wire in the bladder. If you pull on it to make it straight all that happens is that portion of the wire in the ureter comes out first. It is the damnedest thing and the only solution is not to let it happen in the first place. Again, as in the first example, you have to start over which may or may not be easy: i.e. lost access and nephrostomy city.

Rule: Once you have gained access in the ureter be very diligent in not losing it, and often it is assistants trying to help you that end up thwarting your efforts.

When it comes to a scrub tech with "a little urology experience"-watch out. "A little knowledge is indeed a very dangerous thing."

105
That Ain't the Way I Was Trained

"The greater the ignorance, the greater the dogmatism."
Osler

"To unlearn is as hard to learn."
Aristotle

What a worthless response of a physician in defending why he does something a certain way. Is this not the epitome of being dogmatic? This is the way I was trained? Really? Is that all you got?

We were making rounds one day and a resident who had transferred to the Medical College from elsewhere verbalized this reasoning to one of our attendings in defending a procedure the resident had proposed.

The attending says, "So that's the way you were trained huh? So, you are a dog is that right? Can you sit and fetch too?"

I don't really know why doctors use this rationale, but I hear it all the time. In essence, they are saying they are continuing to do something in a way that they were taught years ago. No thinking, no reevaluating, no nothing; just doing it the way they were trained. The other troublesome thing about this excuse and the doctor that would use it is that they don't see how flawed the excuse, and the subsequent execution of it, is.

Rule: Constantly evolve and embrace change. If you catch yourself saying "That is the way I was trained" rethink it. Many physicians tend to be one dimensional and suffer from tunnel vision. Read "Who Moved My Cheese." Which mouse are you?

"And not only are the reactions of patients themselves variable, but we, the doctors, are so fallible, ever beset with the common and fatal facility of reaching conclusions from superficial observations, and constantly misled by the case with which our minds fall into the ruts of one or two experiences."-Osler

106
What's Your Secret?

I am in the OR dressing room changing into scrubs when an older anesthesiologist approaches me and asks a "simple" question.

"How's it going John?"

So, I am very creative when I get this question, because everyone knows most of the responses given in this situation are trite and rhetorical. I am thinking I'll say, "Ed, think of me as a pizza. I am not your normal pizza with eight slices, no Ed, I have sixteen pieces. Which screwed up segment of my life, exactly, are you inquiring about?" But I don't. I did something different. Upon hearing the question I stand up and begin pretending that I am drowning. I extend my face skyward and make an accentuated circle with my mouth and exaggerate attempting to breathe all the while thrashing about my arms as if I am struggling not to sink.

"Well Ed, I am barely above water," I reply breathlessly.

"What's your secret?" he responds.

Rule: Everybody has their own cross to bear, and you really don't know what others are going through just by looking at them. Keep that in mind, won't you?

"Be kind for everyone you meet is fighting a hard battle." -Plato

107
You Are Only as Good as Your Last Case

L et's say that the ebb and flow of your urological life is what waits for you behind the four exam room doors in your office. They are continually filling, emptying, and the content of which is also changing with a myriad of possibilities. On second thought our exam room inhabitants do mirror our own life to a degree.

Monday afternoon: Having done an add on case at noon and missing lunch-

Room One: "Sorry I kept you waiting. How's that circumcision incision doing?" "You cut off way too much skin. When I sit down it disappears. I wouldn't have had this done if I'd known this was going to happen!" "I am sorry you feel that way. You know, the skin of the foreskin does not add to the length of the penis. I only removed the redundant foreskin. The problem may be your supra pubic fat pad that drapes over the penis with sitting." "No, it's not that. You have shortened my penis!"

Room Two: "Sorry I kept you waiting. How are you today?" "I am great. My wife and I cannot express to you enough for saving my life. If you hadn't gotten me into surgery as quickly as you did, and on a weekend, I know I would have died. We have brought you a gift." "A blind hog will find an acorn from time to time," I say.

Room Three: "I am sorry to..." "Your radio station is horrible and it is too loud. I have waited over an hour for you. I should charge *you* for this visit. I had to pay a co-pay for you to biopsy my prostate, a co-pay to get the results, and now another co-pay to see if it has spread. Can I just call for this stuff in the future? I am still getting bills for the hospitalization after the biopsy. Man this is some racket you've got here."

Room Four: "I am so sorry to have kept you waiting. How are things with y'all? "Dr. McHugh we have great news. We're going to have a baby! You did the vasectomy reversal, and a couple of months later we were pregnant. We cannot thank you enough for you and your staff's professional care! If it is a boy, we are going to use your middle name. If all goes well we'll be back for you to do the vasectomy."

Room One Again: "Wow Dr. McHugh. You have really aged. You've got more wrinkles and a lot less hair than the last time I saw you. Are you alright? Is your cancer back?" "I am fine thank you. What brings you our way today?"

Room Two Again: Eighty –year old patient, "Dr. McHugh was your father a urologist? I saw a urologist named McHugh in this complex about twenty years ago." Realizing the patient was referring to me, I respond sadly, "No that was me. You were about sixty and I was about forty. We were both young men back then."

Room Three Again: And on and on and on and on, navigating and enduring the fickle roller coaster ride of vicissitudes that is medical practice.

Rule: Don't rest on your laurels. How patients feel about you is a lot like what they say about the weather in Northeast Georgia: If you don't like it, then stick around; it will change.   Corollary: What have you done for me lately? One other thing: If you are one hour late to the office because of surgery and you have fifteen patients to see that afternoon, well, you are going to be late fifteen times in row and with each patient- an apology to proffer.

"It must be confessed that the practice of medicine among our fellow creatures is often a testy and choleric business."-Osler

108
A Word to the Wise...

Ken Dixon's father was one of the first surgeons of Hall County, Georgia and as a result Ken is an encyclopedia of medical stories. I did not realize until I began this book that most of Ken's stories involve people who are real characters. Recently, he was telling me about a time during his surgical residency at Crawford Long Hospital in Atlanta when he lost his temper with an attending, and that his outburst was witnessed by an older attending standing nearby. Ken, smiling, then said to me, "The guy was abusing me and it was time for it to stop. John, have you ever seen me get mad?"

At this point in telling me this story, it is clear that Ken's memory of the older attending vividly came back to him. He recounted that this particular attending, who he admired very much, would get very close to your face and put a hand on your shoulder while he talked. (They say that LBJ had this habit of speaking to people.) He said that the attending only called people "Pardnuh" or "Chief," and that his philosophy of life came down to two scenarios. For any event or action there were only two consequences: either good would come of it, or only bad would come of it.

After Ken's tirade was completed, the attending called him over and characteristically pulled him close and secured him there with the hand on the shoulder technique. "Pardnuh," he said. "No good can come of that."

The Rotary Four-Way Test:
- Is it the truth?
- Is it fair to all concerned?
- Will it build goodwill and better friendships?
- Will it be beneficial to all concerned?

"Will good or bad come from your words or actions?" Not a bad motto Ken.

Rule: A word to the wise is sufficient.

"A wise man does not need advice and a fool won't take it."

109

The Only Thing ENT Has over Urology is Cocaine

One day in the urology clinic, the intern I have previously mentioned in this book (the one that told the BS-ing older patient that he should treat his impotence by abstaining from sex for six months), was complaining of a head cold.

"I can't breathe. This is miserable."

I had a friend who was the chief resident on ENT, and I arranged for the intern to go to their clinic. Just as an aside, this chief resident knew my older brother from twenty years ago in Columbus, Georgia. He and my brother went to St. Anne-Pacelli Catholic School there. I went there until third grade. I still remember the nuns.

So, the intern goes and about hour later comes back a changed person. I mean, he was showing us how well he could breathe by taking long and exaggerated breaths, and moving around excitedly and seemed really ready to get to work.

"What in the hell did they do to you?" I asked him.

With a big smile and after another demonstrative deep breathe he says, "Cocaine my friend, cocaine."

The ENT boys had put cocaine soaked pledgets in his nose and let it sit for a while and the stuff must have gone systemic.

"Man that was something else. Now I know why people use this stuff. I feel great!"

I had a medical school friend who was telling me about snorting cocaine, and he said he'd do it before going to parties. He says, "I'd do the coke and then go into a room full of people and I felt like King Bad. I loved it."

Rule: If only we could just invent a "cocaine soaked urethral pledget" for the penis. No, that won't work; cocaine is a vasoconstrictor. Never mind.

William Halsted, the father of modern surgery, became addicted to cocaine while experimenting on its use in regional anesthesia.

110
Pee and Run Under It

"Gu Lockett" is how he'd answer the phone in the clinic area of Augusta's VA Hospital Urology Department. Charlie Lockett was Mr. Do It All for anything urology and working with him was a rite of passage for all the urology residents who rotated through "his" department. He was a black urology technician in his late fifties, had gray hair in the style of Albert Einstein, and was a joy to work with.

"Work with the doctor," he'd say as the patient writhed in pain from rigid cystoscopy without sedation. We called it "riding the silver stallion," and you did not want to have that done to you.

Mr. Lockett had all of these idiosyncrasies that I loved. One time he was getting something out of his wallet and I noticed that he had an inordinate volume of bills in it.

"How much money do you have there Mr. Lockett?"

"Probably two thousand."

"My Lord, why so much?"

"You never know what might come up. If you ain't got the money, then the deal might not get done. You got to be ready. Money talks and bullshit walks."

On another occasion, he was attempting to help me get the voiding history of a patient with a language barrier and who was having trouble understanding the terms we were using regarding how he was urinating.

"How do you make your water? You know, your stream. How is your stream? Any trouble voiding?" No response and a look of confusion on the face of the patient.

"Can you pee and run under it?, Mr. Lockett asked.

"Pee and run under it?" I ask. "Where in the hell did you come up with that one?"

"You know doc. When I was young I could pee over a fence post, and I could pee and run under it."

Rule: This phrase has since become my standard of a "good stream."

Definition of a rigid cystoscope: An instrument with a dickhead at both ends.

111
Red Herring

One Saturday morning a friend, who is an anesthesiologist, called me at home. "John, I know you are not on call, but I think my brother has a twisted testicle. I just picked him up at the airport and on the way home in the car he began having acute, extreme pain in his right testicle."

"How old is your brother?" I ask.

"He is thirty-five," he says.

I can hear the brother in the background groaning in pain.

"It would be more likely to be a ureteral stone," I say.

"No John. The pain is in his right testicle. Man he is hurting bad! What should we do? Go to the ER?" he asks.

"Yes and the ER Doc can sort this out. I will call and let them know to be expecting you," I say.

Later that day I called my friend to see how things went at the ER

"They did a scrotal ultrasound with Doppler, and there was blood flow to the testicle so it wasn't torsion. I told them what you said, and they did a CT He had a small ureteral stone that they think he'd already passed, probably in the car going to the ER He's fine now," he says.

Rule: The saying "red herring" is used to describe something that provides a false or misleading clue. It's a hunting phrase from the 1800's which refers to the actions of hunt saboteurs who would drag a smoked herring, which is red in color and strong-smelling, along the hunt route and away from the foxes. This confused the hounds, which were thrown off the scent of the fox to follow, instead, the scent of the red herring.

An occasional prostatism patient will present with dysuria. They will have had antibiotics for presumed prostatitis. Their residual volume will be low and their complaints about the burning mask the true underlying problem; the bladder contracting against an obstructive prostate. If you dodge the red herring of "burning when I pee" and ask about the caliber of stream, you'll find the etiology of the problem as well as its treatment.

112
Watch What You Write and Read What You Sign-Really?

I wouldn't wish on anyone being in a courtroom with twelve jurors, a judge looking on and the prosecuting team brings in a billboard sized rendition of your operative note.

"Dr. McHugh, this is your signature at the end of this operative report, correct?"

"Yes sir."

"So, you read this before you signed it, and you agree with what you wrote?"

This line of questioning revolved around my having stated in the operative report that I advised the gynecologist to do a post-operative IVP and the fact that he had not, and that a ureteral injury was noted two weeks, after discharge.

I answer, "Yes sir, but I don't remember how forcibly I made that recommendation."

Out goes my gargantuan op note and in comes the gynecologist's discharge summary; it is two pages long and takes up a whole wall in the courtroom. In the discharge summary, he dictated that he intended to do an IVP on the patient. An IVP was never ordered by him.

The prosecuting attorney says, "Is this your discharge summary, and is this your signature at the bottom?"

"Yes it is," the gynecologist answers.

"So, you dictated a summary of the hospital stay, you thoroughly read what you dictated and by signing it, you agree with what is here before us. Is that correct?"

"No, sir," he answers.

"I am confused. You signed it. That means you read it, right?"

The gynecologist says, "I am not sure if I read it or not. As a rule I don't read the reports I've dictated. I'd be in medical records all day if I read everything I dictated."

"You are telling the jury that you may have signed this report without having read it?"

"That is correct."

It was brilliant. We are taught all this stuff about documentation, reading what we write, signing only what we have read, but in this case, not having read it was actually protective. "Yes, I signed it but I sign a lot of things without reading it." It left the attorney speechless. I remember thinking how clever the response was. It reminded me of saying, "I don't know" and you are perceived to be more intelligent and wiser.

Do you remember Chauncey Gardner in *Being There*? He speaks in simplistic language to questions and is viewed to be not only brilliant, but clairvoyant.

From *Being There*:

Ron Steigler: Mr. Gardner, uh, my editors and I have been wondering if you would consider writing a book for us, something about your um, political philosophy, what do you say?
Chance the Gardener: I can't write.
Ron Steigler: Heh, heh, of course not, who can nowadays? Listen, I have trouble writing a postcard to my children. Look uhh, we can give you a six figure advance, I'll provide you with the very best ghost-writer, proof-readers...
Chance the Gardener: I can't read.
Ron Steigler: Of course you can't! No one has the time! We, we glance at things, we watch television...
Chance the Gardener: I like to watch TV.
Ron Steigler: Oh, oh, oh sure you do. No one reads!

Rule: If you signed it but didn't read it how can they hold it against you? Brilliant, but ask your attorney about using this technique in your lawsuit when the car-sized op note comes in.

One day at about the time I finished seeing my patients, I was told there was a lawyer that wanted to speak to me. Not knowing any better I spoke to him. He told me he was "on my side" and "all I had done was try to help." He said I was not the focus of those evaluating the lady with the ureteral injury. I liked the guy, we talked about fishing, and I was candid. About six months later I got the news that I was named in the law suit. I came to find out that he represented a class of lawyers who under the guise of helping, go out and speak to potential defendants in a case. My advice to you? If a lawyer comes to your office and asks to speak to you, you are under no obligation to speak to him and you should not speak to him. Burn me once shame on you, burn me twice shame on me. I fell for it, and paid for it; don't you. I saw this lawyer at the trial and asked him why he deceived me. "Doc I had no control over it."

113
Physicians Tend to Fashion a Diagnosis Based on Their Specialty

I treated a friend who happens to be friends with several physicians in our community. He had a proximal uric acid stone that was not visualized on plain films, which, in turn, made ESWL with fluoroscopy problematic. I elected to place a small catheter with a flexible scope and inject contrast on that side and then treat where the contrast stopped. As I was injecting contrast through the catheter I had placed, the anesthesiologist, who also is a friend of the patient, noted that the oxygen saturation was lower than expected for the age and medical condition of our patient. It is easy for the surgeon to know when the anesthesiologist is concerned. Their eyes become fixated on all of the parameters pertaining to the patient and in this case the anesthesiologist was sensing the resistance of the bag in his hand. I was moved by the old-fashioned technique of gauging the resistance.

"What are you thinking?" I said. My worry was that there was infection above the stone and my manipulation has initiated a bacteremia. It has happened to me before, and a patient almost died.

"He's a little tight. I think he'll be alright. I hear wheezes. I'll get a chest x-ray in post op and give him a breathing treatment. The O2 Sat is coming back up."

Another friend, this one a thoracic surgeon, stops by the recovery room and looks at the portable chest x-ray and feels it is relatively clear. However, he says, "I'd put him on Lovenox. I don't think this is an embolus, but it won't hurt to be ahead of it."

When I tell the wife about what happened after the case, she said, "He has gained weight and we are having him checked for sleep apnea." Our patient returned to his room and went home that afternoon with absolutely no sequel to the surgery. Rule: "Medicine is a science of uncertainty and art of probability." -Osler

"There is nothing so stupid as the educated man if you get him off the thing he was educated in."-Will Rogers

114
Surgeon's Motto: Sometimes Wrong but Never in Doubt

Three physicians were duck hunting: an internal medicine doctor, a surgeon, and a pathologist. They were positioned in the above order and about a hundred feet apart.

A group of ducks appeared and approached the position of the internal medicine doctor.

He thinks to himself, "Are these ducks or Canadian geese, or maybe a bird of some sort with a wider wing span?" As he is going through the steps of mental masturbation and contemplating all of the diagnostic possibilities of the types of birds he sees, they pass by him and out of range.

As the ducks approached the surgeon, he begins to fire his gun wildly and in rapid succession. The result is that the majority of the ducks fall dead to the ground in front of him. He and his dog gather all the game and proceed to where the pathologist was stationed.

Throwing all the dead game at the feet of the pathologist, the surgeon says, "Can you tell me what kind of birds these are?"

Rule: If a door of an elevator is closing in front of an internal medicine doctor, he will place his hands in the opening to prevent it from closing. The surgeon will place his head.

"A barber surgeon...is a man who is sufficiently dexterous to wield the razor when he cuts a beard or open an abscess. A person who is skillful with his hands, no more. A performer. As soon as the act extends to the inner organs...instructions and control can come only from the physicians." -William Harvey

115
See One. Do One. Teach One.

I was on a vascular surgery service as a second year surgical intern. The five year urology residency required two years of rotating on all of the surgical specialties. I became friends of most of the chiefs of these various services. It's a funny thing; you do your work, and you will get along fairly well wherever you go. This particular chief and I enjoyed working together, and I learned a lot from him.

On one particular occasion, we were in the intensive care unit and a patient who had just had a tracheostomy placed began having arterial bleeding at the insertion site. About the same time as this was going on, the chief gets a page that his patient was ready for him in the operating room. The patient was to have an above the knee amputation for diabetic vascular disease.

"John. Have you ever done an AKA?" he asks.

"No, I haven't," I say. "I have seen a below the knee amputation though."

"Okay. I want you to go over there and do the amputation," he says as a nurse is prepping the area around the bleeding tracheostomy. He takes out his pen and puts out one of his legs in an exaggerated position in front of the other and begins to draw elliptical lines just above where his knee was. "This is how a fish-mouth incision is made. Once you tie off the arteries and cut the bone, you'll be able to close the skin without tension. You okay with this?"

"Yes, I am comfortable with it. Will I get any grief from the scrub techs when they see me show up without you?"

"Maybe, but here's what you do. After you make the incision ask for a Hummel retractor. When they hear you say that, they'll think you know what the hell you are doing."

Rule: Call me if you need me, but it's a sign of weakness.

This same surgical resident was fond of saying, "Be careful and don't get to cocky John...Dr. Humble just might come to visit!"

Johns Hopkins University was founded in 1876 and the money given to establish it was by Johns Hopkins. Hopkins made his money in the railroad business and retired at the age of fifty-two. His first name was the last name of his paternal great grandmother Margaret Johns. The first president of Johns Hopkins was Daniel Coit Gilman. In time a very talented team of physicians was assembled for the Johns Hopkins University School of Medicine, which was established in 1893. Four of the physicians became known as the "Big Four," pathologist William Welch, surgeon William Halsted, internist William Osler, and gynecologist Howard Kelly. Each of the doctors, in his own way, had a profound and lasting influence on American medical education and research.

Hugh Hampton Young was given a surgical resident spot in 1986 by virtue of another resident leaving. He had no particular interest in urology and in fact was troubled that he was unnoticed by the head of surgery Halsted. Just as he had gotten into the residency program fortuitously, so too, did he begin his illustrious career in urology at Johns Hopkins.

"One day in October, 1897, I was walking rapidly down the long corridor of the hospital. As I turned the corner, I ran into Dr. Halsted with great force and almost knocked him down. I caught him just before he hit the floor and began to apologize profusely. Dr. Halsted, still out of breath, said: 'Don't apologize, Young. I was looking for you, to tell you we want you to take charge of the Department of Genito-Urinary Surgery.' I thanked him and said: 'This is a great surprise. I know nothing about genitourinary surgery.' Whereupon Dr. Halsted replied, 'Welch and I said you didn't know anything about it, but we believe you could learn."- Hugh Hampton Young

Young performed the first perineal prostatectomy in 1904, was the innovator of many the procedures we use today, and is considered, "The father of modern urology."

Considering how Young got his appointment from Halsted, he may have been the first practical example of, "See one, do one, teach one."

116
I Can't See!

Fourth Grade, Columbus, Georgia: My teacher figured out, not me or my family, that I could not see. I remember going down to Pearle Vision with my mother in downtown Columbus. It was a small and narrow shop and at the time, with all the attention I was getting, I felt important and happy to be getting glasses. I remember returning to our home on Flint Drive, getting out of the Ford Falcon station wagon, and seeing the tree across the street that housed our tree house. It was amazing seeing individual leaves. Up until this point I thought all trees from a distance were a mass of green.

From this time, until I was a freshman at North Georgia College in Dahlonega, Georgia, I got a newer and stronger pair glasses every six months. My poor mother would pay five dollars a month in an attempt to stay current with expenses associated with the glasses. I was very nearsighted: Coke-a-cola bottle nearsighted. I learned from experience to refuse any classmate's request to look through my glasses. The resultant knee-jerk response of, "Oh my God, you're blind!" became old and embarrassing very quickly and all future requests denied. Jump ahead to me being a first year urology resident. The strength of my glasses was such that they did not mesh with the lenses in the cystoscope. All I would see when I inserted the scope was blurry red. I thought this was normal. My first cystoscopy at the VA resulted in a bladder perforation and even when this happened I did not know it. It took another resident to figure out what I had done. The fact that I couldn't see became the topic of conversation of all the residents. It was a depressing time for me, as I thought there would be a chance I'd have to choose a new residency.

I stopped attempting doing cystoscopies and would find ways to have someone else do them for me. To my attendings credit, if they knew what was going on with me, they never questioned me about the issue. This was in keeping with Dr. Witherington's overall philosophy of, "It will be all right."

Then I got the idea that maybe the clash between my glasses and the lens of the cystoscope could be corrected by another lens. I got a thirty degree lens and took it down to the ophthalmology department and explained what was going on and thankfully they were very helpful. They tried a series of hand held lens interposed between me and scope and in time we found a power that worked. They gave me this red lens holder that I adapted to the cystoscope. I then found out that Storz made a clip-on device for the scope that you could put the power lens in you needed. (Obviously, this was a problem for others.) So, for three years, I never went anywhere without my clip-on "rectifier." It worked like a charm. That thing saved my career.

After starting private practice, soft contact lenses improved to the point that I could wear them. For some reason, wearing contacts corrected the cystoscope issue. About this time, as well, the flexible cystoscope with an adjustable focus and the use of cameras for the cystoscope made looking directly into the eyepiece obsolete. Today, all of the operating rooms have large adjustable monitors attached to ceiling and hi tech cameras to attach to the scopes making all of the above history moot. So, in the end, it all worked out. Life is funny that way.

Dr. Witherington was right after all: "It will be all right."

Rule: A preacher told a story about a young man who lost his wife and his only son in a car accident. A few years later, the man remarried and had a daughter, and the preacher was able to share this man's journey from hopelessness to happiness. In the preacher's office, he claims as his most prized gift, a piece of wood given to him by the young man with this inscription:

"Your picture has not been completely painted yet."

"You recognize a surgeon or ob-gyn because he has blood on his shoes, the urologist because he has urine on his, and an anesthesiologist because on his you see spots of spilled coffee."-Bernard Cristalli

117

You Don't Cure Strictures, You Manage Them

I have always enjoyed pretending to talk about something completely ridiculous, but in a serious tone, in front of strangers. In fact, on my first trip in an airplane to Washington, D.C., for a Key Club convention, the friend I went with told me, "John, if you don't start acting normal, I am not going to be seen with you."

As a resident I had this "skit" I'd do with the chief resident when we found ourselves in a crowded elevator of patients, residents and employees at Talmadge Hospital. I had a three year old son at the time and the skit involved speaking of him to the chief resident as if my son had gonococcal urethral stricture disease. "Doug, I want to thank you for seeing my son in the clinic today. His stream had gotten down to a dribble and that watering pot perineum of his is making him have to wear diapers again."

"No problem, John. Man, oh man, does he have one bad ass stricture. He's a trooper though; he tolerated an internal urethrotomy in the clinic today like a champ. Y'all can take the catheter out when he stops bleeding. Is he still self-dilating at home with Van Buren sounds?"

"Yes, he is. Well, that is until the 10 French won't go, then his mother uses the filiforms and followers to get him back up to a 16 French. That Blandy you did on him, although I appreciate your efforts, was a lot to go through and then still have to keep up the dilations."

"I understand John, but your son should have thought about all this before he went about catting around. His stricture is pan urethral and very tight. He may end up with s perineal urethrostomy with the stricture he's got."

"Doug, what makes this so hard for his mother and me is that he is only three."

"Well, John, as my mother used to say, 'you make your bed...'

Rule: Gonococcal urethral stricture disease-The gift that keeps on giving.

118
How Much Urine Does a Kidney Make in a Day?

The first malpractice lawsuit that I had the pleasure to endure had to do with a ureteral injury by a gynecologist. I evaluated the patient intraoperatively, saw clear urine efflux from the orifice, and elected not to place a stent. What he had done was fulgurate the ureter and it necrosed in a small area that resulted in an egg-sized urinoma two weeks later. The IVP demonstrating this was lost but there was a report that showed the size and location of the urinoma. I mention this because the prosecuting attorney kept saying, over and over, for the benefit of the jury, "He transected the ureter and this urologist didn't diagnose it!"

Here's something I want to share with you if you find yourself in a courtroom one day. The lawyers use medical terms in which they don't comprehend the nuances of their medical meaning. For instance, that the ureter was damaged is different from "transected." The jury understands "transected" as the complete severing of something; that interpretation is much more egregious than a pinpoint area that allowed for leakage of urine two weeks after the fact. My point is that you know more about urology than your lawyer and the other guy's lawyer and you must be diligent to educate the jury to the correct usage of "our words." (This dawned on me most clearly when I was an expert witness for a fellow urologist years later.)

So, I am witnessing this strategy by the prosecuting attorney, and I ask my team if I can be called to the stand to explain the difference in the terminology and how the course of the patient did not comport with a "transected" ureter.

"When you call me, can I have a board to write on and a magic marker?"

I am called and after the "tell the truth and nothing but the truth" stuff, I ask if I can show the jury something about ureter, explain the x-rays, and why "transected" is giving the wrong impression as to what had happened. The prosecution objects, they approach the judge, they talk and I am given a magic marker and allowed to play teacher. I was so stoked.

We had this big white drawing board that was positioned right in front of the jury and in view of all in the courtroom.

"The IVP done two weeks after the surgery showed a three centimeter collection of urine at the distal left ureter. This small collection of urine however was large enough to impede the flow of urine, and this is the reason the patient had left flank pain in follow up," I say as I am drawing pictures to complement my points.

"The kidneys, depending on how much one drinks, produces about two thousand ccs of urine a day. Obviously, if the ureter had been transected or totally cut in half, there would have been two weeks of urine in the abdomen not just an egg's worth. In addition to this, my intraoperative evaluation revealed urine emanating normally from the ureter. The ureter could not have been, nor was it, transected." Oh, I was good. I remembered Dr. Witherington saying you needed at least a milk carton's worth of a bladder to sleep through the night.

The next day the opposing team's expert witness from St. Louis, no less, and who was not privy to my testimony the day before took the stand.

"Doctor you have testified that in your expert opinion the ureter was transected. How much urine does a kidney make in a day would you say?"

The grandfathered in urogyenecologist did not have an answer and, when pressed, would not estimate.

"You mean to tell me that you have come into our community from some big city up north and have impugned the reputation of one of our board certified urologists and you don't how much urine a kidney makes in a day!"

My attorney in the course of this questioning had started in front of the "expert witness", moved down the line of the front row of jurors and ended standing in front of me with his hands theatrically up in the air. It was a work of art to behold. I was thinking, "This is so cool. This could be a movie. I'm loving this."

After a long pause, the attorney ended with, "That's all I have your honor."

That pretty much did it for me. The next morning my attorney and I met with the judge and I was dismissed on summary judgment. (I still don't know what that phrase means or why it applied to me, but I'm glad it "got me off.") A few days later the jury ruled in favor of the gynecologist.

As an aside, I ran the New York Marathon the weekend between the two weeks of the trial. I didn't have a ticket so I took the subway to a point near the start line and huddled in a group of women who had made a circle to urinate together. When they ran out from the circle, I ran with them back into the flow of the race. Urologists have to be resourceful.

The prosecuting attorney wanted to shake hands when I was dismissed. It wasn't going to happen. Where do they get off with that stuff? What they don't understand (and probably the public for that matter) is how devastating the whole process of a mal practice suit is to a doctor. What is to us is a life altering event for the physician is to them is just another day at work.

Rule: Heads up if you are called into the operating room to help a colleague. If something comes of the case, the attorneys name everyone involved, and you need to at least let that remind you to pursue the most conservative course. I over-thought this one and should have just placed a stent.

My hesitancy in telling others about my prostate cancer and that I probably made a bigger deal out of it than necessary, reminds me of the time I informed my daughter about my first law suit. She was to be the Sugar Plum Fairy in our hometown's ballet company production of the "Nutcracker" and she and her mother were looking at ballet shoes in a magazine. "Bess, I want to tell you that I will be in court all next week for a malpractice lawsuit. One of your friends at school or maybe a teacher may mention or ask you something about it, and it could be in the paper. Daddy has not done anything wrong, it isn't like I could go to jail or anything, it is just something that happens to doctors these days, and it will be O.K." Again, just like my aunt said of my grandfather Robert Cooper Davis, I began to feel the moistness in my eyes beginning; I hate that when it happens. Bess looks at me for a few seconds and then at her mother and says, "Mom, I think I like the pink ones better." It was probably the best thing she could have said.   From "The Decision"

"Lawyers-a profession it is to disguise matters."- Sir Thomas Moore

119
Three Condom Jokes

A man goes into a pharmacy and asks to buy some condoms. The pharmacist sets down a box and says, "That'll be $3.50 plus tax." The man replies, "I don't need the tacks. I'll just roll them on."

A young man goes into a pharmacy and behind the counter is an attractive but older pharmacist. "I'd like to buy some condoms," he says.

"What size?" she asks.

"I don't know."

"Well behind the store we have a fence with holes in it. If you like, you can go back there and measure yourself."

The young man goes around to the back of the store and unbeknownst to him so does the pharmacist. As the young man is measuring himself, she is on the other side of the hole. As he goes down the line trying all the sizes, she does too serving as a receptacle of sorts.

When he is through measuring, he dresses and goes back into the front door of the store and as he does the pharmacist dresses and goes through the back. They arrive at the same time at the counter.

"Well, what size to you want?" she asks.

"The hell with condoms," he says. "I want six feet of that fence!"

What do you call a tire made out of 365 condoms?
A "Goodyear."

Rule: Dysuria and the patient uses condoms? Think latex allergy.

Goodyear Rubber Company developed thin rubber gloves at the request of Dr. William Halsted for his wife Caroline Hampton Halsted. She was a scrub nurse and had mercuric chloride induced dermatitis. The gloves were instituted strictly for her use and had nothing to do with asepsis. It was not until three years later in 1896 that gloves were used for asepsis purposes.

"It is remarkable that during the four or five years, when I was an operator, I wore gloves occasionally, we could be so blind as not to have perceived the necessity for wearing them invariably at the operating table."–William Halsted.

120
Why Do Tigers Bounce?

I had a friend in high school named Weasel who loved to play practical jokes on fellow students. I first became friends with him after he had stuffed wadded up paper above my locker latch making it impossible to open. The locker was destroyed by the shop teacher with a crow bar attempting to get in to it. When I learned who did it, I was so impressed that he became my best friend. In college, despite having all A's, I pretended my entire freshman year that I was failing and on drugs. A math professor assumed that the "Mac" (I was McHugh not McAllister) in the class with a 50 average was me and counseled me about studying. I had a 98 average but when called to the chalk board to do a problem, I'd pretend I did not know the answer.

"I'll work harder sir," I said.

"I hope you will Mac or you'll be going home," my professor would reply.

In medical school I was known for calling my fellow classmates "Bud." I'd say, "How's it going Bud." The word bud became synonymous with John McHugh. So one day in our lecture hall of about two hundred students, we are learning the embryology of the liver. The professor must have said a hundred times, the term "liver bud" in describing the development of the liver. I couldn't stand it. I raise my hand and I am recognized.

"What is the precursor to the development of the liver, Bud?" I asked emphasizing the word "Bud." The entire class erupted in laughter much to the puzzlement of the professor. I was elected class president the next year in large part from people knowing me from remarks like this.

During residency, in a crowded elevator I pretended that I had gonorrhea and that I was treating it with a roll of "Cipro mints" that a Cipro drug representative had given all the residents.

Outside the elevator an intern, who I had asked if he felt he needed one too, stops me and asks, "Dr. McHugh, why do you f*** with people all the time?"

"Do you know why Tiggers bounce?" I ask in return.

"No, I don't"
"Because, that is what Tiggers do best!"

Rule: Well, I gotta go now. I've got a lotta bouncin' to do! Hoo-hoo-hoo-hoo! T-T-F-N: ta-ta for now!-Tigger

121
The Heat of Battle-The Fog of War

A general on a horse, at a high vantage point, is observing an ongoing battle with members of his staff and reporters from his home country. "General," one of the reporters asks, "why do you wear such a bright crimson jacket? Does that not make you more of a target for the sharpshooter?"

"I wear this color because in the event I am shot, the blood will not be noticeable to my men. I do not want to alarm them as it might affect their confidence to fight the enemy."

At that moment a bullet whizzes by and grazes the lower lobe of the general's left ear, missing his head by less than an inch.

After a moment the general says, "Sargent, fetch me my brown trousers."

I have a son who is an Eagle Scout, and I have received what is often referred to as "A masters in scouting," the Wood Badge. I mention this to make this point; there is a huge difference in asking a scout to start a fire vs. asking a scout to start a fire in three minutes with only three matches. Limits on time and resources accelerate the stress, likelihood for failure and influences decision making. Think about the quarterback who has at best five seconds to read the defense and decide which route he is going choose while massive defensive linemen close in to tackle him.

So, for a fellow physician to come in the next morning and judge an action a fellow physician pursued the night before while in the heat of battle is, at the very least, unfair. To me, the doctors who judge, just as those who would judge anyone else speaks volumes. They are, in a cheap way, attempting to elevate themselves while at the same time diminish a fellow "warrior." Recognize it for what it is, and then after noting, don't you do this to others. Do unto others as...you know the drill.

Rule: If you weren't there, it is probably best not to judge.

"Never let your tongue say a slighting word of a colleague."-Osler

122
Don't Eat the Yellow Snow

A fter Christmas dinner a husband and wife are at the kitchen window washing dishes. As the husband hands a dish to his wife he says, "I think I am going to have to speak to Susan's boyfriend." "Why is that?" the wife asks.

"Well, look out there. His name has been peed in the snow," the husband says.

"Ah, honey. Don't be so hard on the young man. You did that type of thing yourself many times when you were younger," the wife replies.

"Yeah, that's true. The problem is that his name is in our daughter's handwriting!

You remember Frank Zappa don't you? Believe it or not, I had an album of his in seventh grade that my older brother forgot to take back to school with him. There is a clip of Zappa on the Johnny Carson show playing a bicycle; he was symbolic of an era of progressive music and sounds. His song "Don't Eat the Yellow Snow" is an iconic creation by him.

Zappa was diagnosed with prostate cancer at age fifty and was dead three years later. If you want to see something poignant, watch his last interview. He says in that interview, which is on YouTube, he doesn't understand how he could have a cancer that is not curable with surgery. It's a good question, and, unfortunately, a question that is still being asked today. Learning of his death from prostate cancer years after I had finished residency was really the first time I realized the dual nature of prostate cancer. So when your patient asks, "Prostate cancer is the slow growing type ain't it?" Just remember Zappa.

Rule: Let Frank Zappa's death as a young man in the prime of his creative life be a reminder to you, and your patients, of the "Frank Zappa kind" of prostate cancer. No male should leave your office without an accounting of the rectal exam.

"One finger in the throat and one in the rectum makes a good diagnostician." -Osler

123
Doctors, Pigs, and Incrementalism

incrementalism (noun): A policy or advocacy of a policy of political or social change by degrees: gradualism.

I was thinking about all of the intrusions into the lives and the profession of physicians by the government, insurance companies and hospitals and this joke came to mind. Most everything reminds me of a joke.

An insurance salesman is approaching a house that he intends to call on and notices in the side yard a three legged pig. He knocks on the door, introduces himself and after talking about insurance for a while, asks the man of the house about the pig.

"So, tell me about that pig you have in your yard. Why does it only have three legs?"

"Oh that pig is very special. Our house caught on fire one night about a year ago and we were all asleep when it happened. That pig realized it and ran through the house oinking real loud to wake everybody up and get them out of the house. He saved the lives of my entire family. That's one smart pig he is," says man.

"So, he has only three legs. Did he lose one in the fire saving y'all?" the salesman asks.

"Nooooo," the man says, "a pig that special you don't eat all at one time."

Rule: Yeah, us doctors are real special too. They ain't gonna eat us either. At least, not all at one time.

Will Rogers said one time: "Be glad you ain't getting all the government you pay for."

If he were alive today he's say: "Be glad you ain't getting all the government health care you pay for."

124
Homonyms, Synonyms, Eponyms, Euphemisms, Aphorisms, Proverbs-Oh My!

Homonyms: Words that have a similar sound.
- Emergency room: "Momma cut her hand and we had to take her to the mushroom."
- Intensive Care Unit: "Daddy got so sick they had to put him in the expensive care unit".
- Prostate gland: "I hurt in my prospect gland."
- Tetanus shot: "I stepped on a nail and had to get a technical shot."
- Urologist: Urineologist
- Dr. McHugh: Dr. DickHuge
- Urinary retention: McHurinary retention

Synonyms: Words that have similar meanings. Synonyms for aphorism- maxim, axiom, proverb, saying, adage, gnome, epigram, dictum, saw, etc. Synonyms for urologists:
- Captain of the stream team
- Penis machinist
- Phallic mechanic
- Dick Doctor
- Pecker checker
- A doctor that works "below the belt."

Euphemism: A mild, vague or indirect term for one considered more blunt or offensive.
- A euphemism for having sex would be "love making" or "sleep with."

Judge to man on trial for soliciting a prostitute: "Sir, did you *sleep* with this woman?"
"Not a wink your honor."

Eponym: The person for which something, such as a disease, is named.

- Throckmorton sign: As seen on a KUB, the penis points to side of the pathology; it is correct almost fifty percent of the time.

Proverbs: A short pithy saying in frequent and widespread use that expresses a basic truth or practical precept.

- Proverbs 12:15- The way of fools seems right to them, but the wise listen to advice. (Not a bad admonition for the urological resident to listen to their attendings. Remember, you have the rest of your career to do it your way and on "your dime.")

Axiom: A self-evident truth that requires no proof.

- Circumcision: You can take from it but you can't add to it.
- I can explain it to you but I can't understand it for you.
- He who has five and spends six has no need for a purse.
- Nothing is impossible to the man who doesn't have to do it.
- The man that trots around will find a bone.
- When there is work to do Nature sends in the blood vessels.
- When you point your finger at someone there are three pointing back at you.
- The only time you should look down on someone is to help them up.
- He who has a broad tongue often has a narrow mind.
- Whether you think you can or you can't-you're right.
- Before you embark on a journey of revenge, dig two graves.
- If a disease has several options for treatment then there is no one good one.
- "Beware of the men that call you Doc. They rarely pay their bills."-Osler.
- Be kind to the child with enuresis; even the lowliest of animals will not sleep in their own urine.

125
Blueberries, PSA, the Flag and the Greatest Generation

I removed the prostate of a man who had a farm with numerous blueberry bushes. He enjoyed picking them by the quart to sell and to give away. It was my good fortune to be one of the special people with whom he shared his blueberries. He would knock on the back door of my office and then enter with several fruit baskets of blueberries. They were always packed so nicely, gorgeous, no stems and washed. He never called to let me know he was coming but I'd always stop to say thank you and to eat several handfuls.

After several years of getting my early summer batch of blueberries, he said to me, "Doc, I'm not selling them anymore. It ain't worth $3.25 a quart to pick them." This made me feel all the more special.

Interesting thing about this guy, his PSA after the prostatectomy gradually climbed up to 2.5. As it trended upward, I'd ask him about seeing a radiation therapist to treat "the bed" of the prostate. Each time he'd decline and I'd see him again in six months.

Then a funny thing happened; the PSA stopped going up. We must have checked for years at six month intervals and there was absolutely no change above the 2.5. I had never seen this phenomena before then and I have not seen it since; "When all else fails, listen to the patient."

After about fifteen years of working with this patient, he died of another problem and his family asked if I'd be a pallbearer. I was flattered and moved by the gesture. He was a veteran of WWII and it was to be a military funeral. Have you ever been to one? My mother was a veteran of the Coast Guard and we could have gotten an American Flag for her service but things happened so fast, we never requested one. Getting her flag is on my bucket list of things to do one day.

He died in winter as I recall and the day of the funeral was overcast, cold and misty. I remember that the graveyard looked exactly how one would be depicted in movie, a somber atmosphere matching the dreariness of the occasion. I remember seeing the grave diggers about a hundred yards away near a backhoe awaiting their turn. At the grave site there were two veteran soldiers in dress uniforms; one with a triangular folded American flag, the other with a bugle and both standing at crisp attention. Their appearance and demeanor embodied a gesture of the utmost respect. I forget the timing of things but "Taps" was played at one point and the flag was ceremoniously given to the widow. It was a very beautiful ceremony and conjured memories of my mother having been in the Coast Guard and thoughts about "the greatest generation." The whole scene was overwhelming.

The nicest and luckiest thing about the timing of my career is that I have had the honor of working with World War II veterans. I have had several patients who landed on D-Day. I have one who was involved in every battle in the Pacific and was preparing for the assault on Japan when he got the news of the atomic bomb. (He didn't have an issue with Truman's using it.) One patient was wounded on Christmas Eve during the Battle of the Bulge. He was a machine gun operator and said, "Other than people shooting at me, it was the prettiest day in the snow I have ever seen." I have a ninety plus year old patient who flew "The Hump." (The eastern portion of the Himalayan Mountains over which airmen flew transport planes from India to China. Almost six hundred planes were lost and 1659 personnel were lost or reported missing.)

Another veteran has over 350 jumps and constant arthritic pain as a result. I asked him the question, "Why would you jump out of a perfectly good airplane?"

He said, "That's the deal. They weren't any good airplanes!"

This patient told me as well that, "I told the commander that the plane we were in needed repairs and new parts. He told me that they were not going to repair the plane and not to worry about its condition; we were going to be jumping out of it anyway."

I love history and have read many of the books on World War II, regarding both the European and Pacific theaters, and this made each of the interactions with these heroes even more special.

So, how to end this story from a "urological perspective?" let's see. In the Battle of the Bulge I referenced earlier, the American troops were surrounded by the Germans and in a desperate situation. The German commander sent an envoy to demand surrender by the Americans or they would face "certain destruction." The American commander, General McAuliffe, famously responded with one word, "Nuts."

Rule: If you have the opportunity to see a War World II vet, take a minute to inquire about and thank them for their service. Each of their stories is truly fascinating. They may very well have on a hat that denotes their theater of service. They will appear very old and most probably accompanied by a family member and a walker. Don't let this deceive you, they are American heroes. A pathology professor at the Medical College, Dr. Teabeaut, used to say, putting a finger to his temple, "You have to use your 'mind's eye' to see some things." Listen to "Veronica" by Elvis Costello.

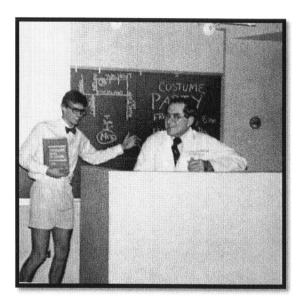

The author as a medical student singing "I'm in the Mood for Love" to Dr. J. Robert Teabeaut in front of the sophomore class lecture hall. That's a hand tied bow tie and pink boxer shorts my friend...pretty spiffy.

Resources

Aequanimitas. William Osler. P. Blakiston's Son and Co. 1910.

Aphorisms and Quotations for the Surgeon. Moshe Schein. tfm Publishing Limited. 2003.

Aphorisms. Hippocrates. Kessinger Publishing, LLC. 2010.

Geary's Guide to the World's Great Aphorisms. James Geary. Bloomsbury. 2007.

Medical Axioms, Aphorisms, and Clinical Memoranda. James Alexander Lindsay. H.K. Lewis and Co. LTD. 1923.

Osler. Charles S. Bryan, M.D. Oxford University Press. 1997. Sir William Osler: Aphorisms from His Bedside Teaching and Writing. Henry Schuman. 1950.

Sir William Osler Aphorisms from His Bedside Teachings and Writings, Sir William Osler, William Bennett Bean, Henry Schuman, 1950.

The Art of War. Sun Tzu. Filiquarian Publishing, LLC. 2006.

The Decision: Your Prostate Biopsy Shows Cancer. Now What? John McHugh M.D. Jennie Cooper Press. 2010.

The Journals of Lewis and Clark. John Bakeless. First Signet Printing. 2002.

The Quotable Osler. Mark Silverman MD, T. Jock Murray MD, Charles S. Bryan MD. American College of Physicians. 2003.

The Viking Book of Aphorisms. W. H. Auden and Louis Kronenberger. Dorset Press. 1962.

William Stewart Halsted: A Lecture by Dr. Peter D. Olch, J Scott Rankin, Ann Surg. 2006 March; 243(3): 418–425

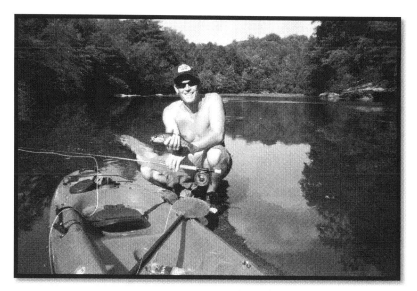

Chattahoochee River above Duncan Bridge

"A bad day fishing is better than a good day at work...any day."

Made in the USA
Charleston, SC
30 April 2015